P9-DBH-859

THE EVERYTHING

HEALTH GUIDE TO

ADULT ADD/ADHD

Dear Reader,

Adult attention deficit hyperactivity disorder (ADHD) affects the lives of millions of adults. We hope you will find this book a helpful and informative resource, whether you are an ADHD adult yourself, know someone who is, or are curious to learn more about the disorder.

Although no one knows exactly what causes adult ADHD and there is currently no cure, rapid advances in technology are leading to more effective diagnostic and treatment modalities. Unfortunately, only a small percentage of adults with ADHD are ever diagnosed and treated because diagnostic criteria for adults are based on childhood ADHD symptoms. Because of this, many untreated adults believe their adult ADHD symptoms are personal flaws. Fortunately, researchers are currently pushing for the creation of adult ADHD criteria that would greatly facilitate the diagnosis of adult ADHD.

Today, most ADHD adults who receive appropriate treatment lead happy, productive lives. In fact, many ADHD adults have achieved great fame and fortune and made lasting contributions to society.

Hopefully, this guide will inform and inspire ADHD adults and their loved ones about a wide range of issues regarding the disorder and affect their lives in a positive way.

Carole Jacobs
Isadore Wendel, PhD

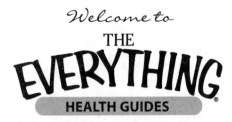

Welcome to

THE
EVERYTHING

HEALTH GUIDES

Everything® Health Guides are a part of the bestselling *Everything*® series and cover important health topics like anxiety, postpartum care, and thyroid disease. Packed with the most recent, up-to-date data, *Everything*® Health Guides help you get the right diagnosis, choose the best doctor, and find the treatment options that work for you. With this one comprehensive resource, you and your family members have all the information you need right at your fingertips.

 Alerts

Urgent warnings

 Facts

Important snippets of information

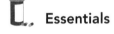 **Essentials**

Quick handy tips

When you're done reading, you can finally say you know **EVERYTHING**®!

PUBLISHER Karen Cooper

DIRECTOR OF ACQUISITIONS AND INNOVATION Paula Munier

MANAGING EDITOR, EVERYTHING® SERIES Lisa Laing

COPY CHIEF Casey Ebert

ACQUISITIONS EDITOR Katrina Schroeder

ASSOCIATE DEVELOPMENT EDITOR Elizabeth Kassab

SENIOR DEVELOPMENT EDITOR Brett Palana-Shanahan

EDITORIAL ASSISTANT Hillary Thompson

EVERYTHING® SERIES COVER DESIGNER Erin Alexander

LAYOUT DESIGNERS Colleen Cunningham, Elisabeth Lariviere, Ashley Vierra, Denise Wallace

Visit the entire Everything® series at *www.everything.com*

THE EVERYTHING® HEALTH GUIDE TO ADULT ADD/ADHD

Expert advice to find the right diagnosis, evaluation, and treatment

Carole Jacobs and Isadore Wendel, PhD, MSCP

Foreword by Theresa Cerulli, MD

adamsmedia
Avon, Massachusetts

616.8589
JAC

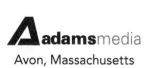

Copyright © 2010 by F+W Media, Inc.
All rights reserved. This book, or parts thereof, may not be reproduced in any form without permission from the publisher; exceptions are made for brief excerpts used in published reviews.

An Everything® Series Book.
Everything® and everything.com® are registered trademarks of F+W Media, Inc.

Published by Adams Media, a division of F+W Media, Inc.
57 Littlefield Street, Avon, MA 02322 U.S.A.
www.adamsmedia.com

ISBN 10: 1-60550-999-X
ISBN 13: 978-1-60550-999-0

Printed in the United States of America.

10 9 8 7 6 5 4 3 2 1

Library of Congress Cataloging-in-Publication Data
is available from the publisher.

This publication is designed to provide accurate and authoritative information with regard to the subject matter covered. It is sold with the understanding that the publisher is not engaged in rendering legal, accounting, or other professional advice. If legal advice or other expert assistance is required, the services of a competent professional person should be sought.

—From a *Declaration of Principles* jointly adopted by a Committee of the American Bar Association and a Committee of Publishers and Associations

Many of the designations used by manufacturers and sellers to distinguish their products are claimed as trademarks. Where those designations appear in this book and Adams Media was aware of a trademark claim, the designations have been printed with initial capital letters.

The Everything® Health Guide to Adult ADD/ADHD is intended as a reference volume only, not as a medical manual. In light of the complex, individual, and specific nature of health problems, this book is not intended to replace professional medical advice. The ideas, procedures, and suggestions in this book are intended to supplement, not replace, the advice of a trained medical professional. Consult your physician before adopting the suggestions in this book, as well as about any condition that may require diagnosis or medical attention. The author and publisher disclaim any liability arising directly or indirectly from the use of this book.

This book is available at quantity discounts for bulk purchases.
For information, please call 1-800-289-0963.

All the examples and dialogues used in this book are fictional, and have been created by the author to illustrate medical situations.

Acknowledgments

Thanks to Katrina Schroeder at Adams Media, Robert G. DiForio at D4E0 Literary Agency, and attorney Tim Whisman for his expertise on Social Security Disability Insurance for ADHD adults. Thanks also to psychologist Harold Burke, PhD, MSCP, for his expertise on neurofeedback.

Contents

Foreword

There are more than 8 million adults in the United States who have attention deficit hyperactivity disorder (ADHD), but only 10 to 15 percent of them have been diagnosed and treated. Despite media accounts to the contrary, ADHD is still significantly underdiagnosed in both children and adults. The heartbreaking result of this neglect is that we are missing the opportunity to help millions of people suffering from this very treatable condition.

The Everything® Health Guide to Adult ADD/ADHD provides something for everyone. You may have a friend or family member who has been diagnosed with ADHD, you may have ADHD yourself, or you may be questioning whether the symptoms you struggle with daily are due to undiagnosed ADHD. You may simply be drawn to this fascinating glimpse of how the brain works to focus, pay attention, organize, file, and store information.

I feel privileged to work in neuropsychiatry, a field that is growing rapidly as science uncovers the mysteries of the mind. I have been specializing in ADHD for more than ten years, and continue to be amazed at how much new information has surfaced in this relatively short span of time. As you read this book, Carole Jacobs and Isadore Wendel will take you on a remarkable journey to understanding ADHD—where we began, the state of today's science, and where we are going.

What is ADHD? The name of this condition has changed over the years, and so has the way we define it. ADHD is the most common neurobiological childhood condition. It affects 7 percent of school-age children worldwide and 4 percent of adults. It is strongly genetic—more easily inherited than breast cancer, asthma, and even schizophrenia. The heritability factor for ADHD is .77, which means if you have been diagnosed with ADHD there is a 77 percent chance you have the condition simply because you inherited it. The days of blaming bad parenting for a medical condition are hopefully numbered.

As a specialist in ADHD, I'm often asked if I get bored seeing "just ADHD" patients. I get a chuckle when I hear this since my ADHD patients are usually the ones keeping me on my toes. In fact, ADHD exists alone only 30 percent of the time; far more often there are conditions that co-occur with ADHD such as depression, anxiety, tic disorders, bipolar disorder, learning disabilities, and substance abuse. Jacobs and Wendel skillfully address the challenge of accurately diagnosing ADHD and the co-existing conditions while ruling out all the other medical and psychological disorders that present with ADHD-like symptoms.

We all have the ability to increase awareness, share accurate information, educate others, dispel the myths, and improve the quality of care and support for individuals with ADHD. It is my hope that you will integrate the information from this book into your everyday lives and spread the word on adult ADHD. I believe you will find the book to be a well-organized, comprehensive, and thought-provoking text you can refer to time and again. It has been a pleasure to introduce you to *The Everything® Health Guide to Adult ADD/ADHD* and become part of your journey.

Theresa Cerulli, MD

Introduction

We all have days when we can't find our keys, always seem to say the wrong thing at the wrong time, or just can't seem to complete anything we start. But for adults with attention deficit hyperactivity disorder (ADHD), these days can be the norm rather than the exception.

Many people have symptoms of adult ADHD but don't realize that what they're feeling is a legitimate condition with promising treatments. They may feel hopeless, worthless, and bored without reason. They may be easily distracted and impulsive. They may be so disorganized and forgetful that their condition has unraveled every area of their lives, from job performance to personal relationships.

Contrary to popular belief, ADHD is not a condition found only in children. Although the disorder is more common in children, millions of adults also suffer from it.

Unfortunately, only 15 percent of adults who have ADHD are ever diagnosed or treated. One factor fueling the silent epidemic of adult ADHD is that adults continue to be diagnosed on criteria that were developed for children with the disorder, which do not accurately reflect the condition's effects on adults.

In addition, many adults struggle for years with undiagnosed adult ADHD and simply don't realize they are affected by a condition that can be diagnosed and treated. For those who do seek help, getting a correct diagnosis can be complicated by the overlap between the symptoms of adult ADHD and many other common psychiatric conditions, including clinical depression, anxiety, obsessive compulsive disorder, and bipolar disorder.

Many undiagnosed adults rely on a variety of coping mechanisms to deal with their symptoms, sometimes risking their health or even their lives in an attempt to appear "normal." It's not unusual for adults with ADHD to work many hours of overtime to keep up with colleagues or to stay up all night studying for a test their classmates easily prepared for in an hour.

To mask symptoms of inattention, drowsiness, anxiety, and depression, many sufferers also abuse alcohol and illegal stimulant drugs. Some become so adept at hiding symptoms that their family, friends, and physicians never suspect they have a problem until the situation becomes impossible to ignore.

Most adults with ADHD suffer highly chaotic lives as they struggle daily with concomitant problems ranging from poor sleeping habits and high risk behavior to associated psychiatric conditions including depression, drug abuse, and learning disabilities. Erratic work performance accounts for billions of dollars in lost earnings.

This health guide offers practical advice on the telltale signs and symptoms of adult ADHD and information on getting a reliable diagnosis, evaluation, and treatment. It may also help remove years of blame, shame, and guilt by reassuring you that you're not really a collection of your symptoms (lazy, crazy, stupid, careless, dishonest), but rather the victim of a neurobiological syndrome whose symptoms can be treated.

By reading this book, you'll also glean the basic medical knowledge necessary to talk intelligently to your doctor about your condition. You'll learn about the condition's classic symptoms, new diagnostic and evaluation techniques, and an increasingly sophisticated arsenal of high-tech treatment and medication modalities used to treat the condition.

It's not easy for an adult to live with ADHD. But the good news is that most adults with ADHD can be successfully diagnosed and treated and go on to lead more productive lives. The key to getting and staying well is knowledge. By picking up this book, you've made a commitment to learn as much as you can about adult ADHD and taken the first step in your journey to improved health and happiness.

CHAPTER 1

Learning the Basics

Not so long ago, attention deficit disorder (ADD), which is now called attention deficit hyperactivity disorder (ADHD), was a disorder experts believed was limited to children. The conventional wisdom was that kids grew out of the condition sometime during puberty and that symptoms did not continue into adulthood. Today, however, experts know that while ADHD begins in childhood, many people continue to have the disorder as adults. In fact, research now shows that 4 percent of the adult population suffers from ADHD—a total of more than 8 million people.

Origin and History

In 1902, Dr. G. F. Still, a researcher who worked with children with behavior disorders, theorized that the behavior problems were the result of neurological problems, not bad parenting. For the next six decades, researchers used neurological testing to search the brain for structural abnormalities that might explain the symptoms.

During the 1970s, researchers began looking more closely at symptoms of hyperactivity and concluded that the disorder appeared to be caused by cognitive disabilities of memory and attention problems. Around this time, scientists also discovered that attention problems could exist without hyperactivity and were likely to persist into adulthood.

The Mysterious Condition Finally Gets a Name

In the mid-1970s, ADHD was finally classified as an official disorder. Studies around this time showed the condition appeared to be highly genetic. Many parents of children with ADHD also suffered from the telltale signs of ADHD, including inattention, impulsivity, and hyperactivity. But the adults were manifesting their ADHD symptoms differently.

Today, scientists agree that ADHD is a biological disorder of the nervous system that begins in children and often continues into adulthood. While the jury is still out on the exact cause of the condition, studies increasingly point to a chemical imbalance in three of the brain's key neurotransmitters—dopamine, norepinephrine, and serotonin.

How ADD Became ADHD

To cover their bases, psychiatrists decided in 1980 to reclassify ADHD as two separate subsets. One was attention deficit disorder with hyperactivity, or ADD – H. The other was attention deficit disorder without hyperactivity, or ADD no H. On further study, researchers realized hyperactivity/impulsivity was actually a larger problem than inattention, and decided to change the name of the disorder to reflect their findings.

In 1987, the disorder was renamed attention deficit hyperactivity disorder, or ADHD, and reclassified as a disorder with not two, but three distinct subsets: inattentive, hyperactive/impulsive, and combination (people who display both inattentive and hyperactive/impulsive symptoms). For the purpose of this book, the disorder will be called adult ADHD to comply with current psychiatric terminology.

Adult ADHD: A Silent Disorder

Getting a diagnosis for adult ADHD can be a difficult and time-consuming process. One reason is that the disorder has as many faces as people who suffer from it and so very few people fit into the tidy classic diagnosis established by the American Psychiatric Association. Often, a parent doesn't realize she has ADHD until her child is diagnosed with the condition and she realizes she has many of the same symptoms.

Essential

According to new genetic studies, one reason it may be so difficult to diagnose adult ADHD is that it is probably not just one disorder. Instead, it's likely to be a cluster of slightly different disorders, each one of which may have its own causes, diagnoses, and treatments.

In addition, the manifestation of core symptoms of ADHD change dramatically as a person moves from childhood to adolescence to adulthood. For instance, perhaps both you and your child have trouble focusing and paying attention, or perhaps you and your child are both restless and at times reckless. In both cases, the two of you are likely to manifest your symptoms in much different ways. As you examine your past behavior, you may begin to see a common thread between your difficulties with playmates on the school playground and your problems relating to your colleagues at work.

The Hidden ADHD Epidemic in Females

Throughout the history of ADHD, research has focused almost exclusively on men. In fact, until the 1990s scientists believed ADHD was a rarity in females, affecting only one female for every nine males. Today, the ratio has been narrowed to one woman

3

for every two men. Exciting new research is finally untangling the mysteries of how ADHD affects adult women, what causes it, what it looks like, how it differs from the condition in men, and why it has remained an invisible disorder until just recently.

In many cases, researchers failed to notice that many females were also suffering from ADHD simply because their symptoms did not manifest in the same ways. Boys and men with the disorder tend to be aggressive, hostile, and occasionally violent, exhibiting the sort of behavior that gets you put in the corner in grade school, in trouble with the law in your teens, and fired from a job as an adult.

On the other hand, girls and women with ADHD rarely manifest the loud, angry, hostile behavior exhibited by boys their age. Instead, they tend to be shy and a little spacey, although those are just two of the many ways females manifest ADHD differently than men. Here are some of the major ADHD symptoms in girls and women.

❑ Women tend to blame themselves for having the disorder and turn their depression and anxiety inward, while men are more likely to rage against society or exhibit hostile or violent behavior.

❑ Hormonal swings in women are highly likely to exacerbate symptoms of adult ADHD in women. Unfortunately, they are often written off as symptoms of premenstrual syndrome (PMS), pregnancy, or menopause.

❑ Studies show that teenage girls with ADHD suffer more from peer pressure and rejection than boys do, possibly because girls may put a higher priority on being accepted by their peers than boys.

❑ Women with ADHD typically have a lot more trouble expressing their anger than men do, and they tend to take it out on themselves rather than on society.

❑ Many careers that are traditionally considered to be the domain of women are not very friendly to women with ADHD.

For instance, teachers and nurses must be organized, detail-oriented, and able to meet important deadlines—skills that many women with ADHD find difficult to master. Being a housewife can be equally overwhelming, especially if a woman has to manage the bulk of the household chores, finances, and child care duties.

❑ More women than men with adult ADHD are single parents, and more than half of women with ADHD are raising at least one child with the disorder.

❑ Research shows that women with adult ADHD get less support and acceptance from husbands than women give husbands with the condition.

The Accidental Diagnosis

Studies show that three out of four adults diagnosed with ADHD are also suffering from associated conditions like anxiety and depression. Many adults first learn they have adult ADHD when they seek medical help for depression or anxiety and learn that these conditions are the symptoms of a far more complicated disorder.

The Problem with Overlapping Conditions

Getting the right diagnosis can also be complicated by the overlap between the symptoms of adult ADHD and the symptoms of other common psychiatric conditions, such as clinical depression and anxiety. In addition, many undiagnosed adults have found ways to "live with" adult ADHD so it doesn't disrupt their lives. They learn how to mask the symptoms so well that their family physicians never suspect they have the disorder.

Differences Between Childhood and Adult ADHD

While few studies have tracked the progress of ADHD from childhood into adulthood, researchers do know that some basic symptoms of ADHD change as you age. Some symptoms, such as hyperactivity, restlessness, agitated behavior, and the need to move or make excessive noise, tend to fade. Others, such as chronic disorganization, the inability to plan or prioritize, and the inability to meet deadlines, tend to get worse.

Why ADHD Is More Serious in Adults

Adult ADHD impacts every area of an adult's life, from his ability to make a living to his chances for a happy marriage and family. Because of the all-encompassing nature of the condition, experts believe it is far more serious and life-threatening than the childhood version of the disorder.

Essential

One hallmark symptom of adult ADHD is an inability to self-regulate. This affects a wide range of things, from your ability to perform tasks and jobs to your ability to organize and prioritize at work and at home so you can remember to get things done and plan for the future.

As a child, you might have engaged in such risky behavior as doing wheelies around the playground on your tricycle. But as an adult, your risky speed-demon habits could be potentially deadly to yourself and others. This is particularly true if they include such activities as flying down a black diamond slope at a ski resort before you've mastered the snow plow. Racing through a project at work without reading the fine print, and getting fired as a result, is another way that reckless behavior can seriously impact an adult. In addition, risky behavior can be lethal to your financial health if it involves gambling away your last dime in Las Vegas or investing all your savings with a fly-by-night scheme.

Unfortunately, reckless behavior is just one of many adult ADHD symptoms that have the potential to sabotage an adult's life. A child's impulsiveness might translate into demanding that Mommy give her a dish of ice cream right now. In an adult, it could translate into impulsive behavior like unprotected sex, drug or alcohol abuse, or quitting a job without a back-up plan. A child's attention problems might result in getting a bad grade on a homework paper. But an adult who zones out during an important business meeting could lose the contract—or even her job.

You Can Run but You Can't Hide

As you can probably imagine, living with adult ADHD is like trying to tame a three-ring circus. Many adults, especially those who have not been diagnosed or treated, will go to great lengths to disguise or cope with the symptoms of the disease.

Some compensate for feeling like social outcasts by drowning out their feelings with drugs or alcohol, and this can lead to other long-term health issues. Others try to cope with their inability to complete projects or get things done on time by making excuses, or by passing their work off to others. For many reasons, the behavior of adults with ADHD often alienates others and turns sufferers in loners, hermits, and social misfits.

📋 Fact

Many people don't know what defines adult ADHD behavior. True ADHD symptoms are long-term and severe enough to impair everyday functioning. They also must occur in more than one environment—at work, at home, and in social settings.

All too often, adults with severe cases of undiagnosed ADHD decide it's easier to give up than get better. Some decide to live on the fringes of society, while others hop from one menial job to another, choosing low-paying jobs over work that would tap their substantial brain power but also expose them to criticism and failure.

Debunking the Myths

Although the exact cause or causes of ADHD remains unknown, advances in research throughout the years have ruled out a number of myths about the disorder. Unfortunately, many continue to exist even without scientific backing. Here are a few of the most common misconceptions you may encounter.

Myth: Adult ADHD is not a real disorder, but a way for deadbeats to excuse laziness, a lack of motivation, or alcoholism or drug abuse.

Fact: Scientific research over the last hundred years has consistently identified people who suffer from impulsivity, an inability to concentrate and focus, and hyperactivity. Today, the condition is officially recognized by many federal agencies and organizations, including the U.S. Department of Education, the Office for Civil Rights, the U.S. Congress, the National Institutes of Health (NIH), and major professional medical, psychiatric, psychological, and educational associations.

Myth: ADHD is caused by a lack of discipline in the home.

Fact: Research shows that being stricter with children with ADHD only makes them worse. Experts say it is counterproductive to use discipline to correct the condition of a child whose biological disease causes a lack of self-control.

Myth: It's not possible to accurately diagnose ADHD.

Fact: Although no single medical test can diagnose ADHD, physicians use a combination of evaluations, interviews, and medical tests to diagnose the disorder with a high degree of certainty.

Myth: Adult ADHD is caused by brain injury.

Fact: Although some people who have been in accidents exhibit signs of behavior similar to adult ADHD, research shows that only a small percentage of adults with ADHD have actually suffered traumatic brain injuries.

Myth: Consuming too much sugar can cause adult ADHD.

Fact: Recent studies show no correlation between sugar consumption and adult ADHD. However, eating excessive amounts of sugar can exacerbate hyperactivity in some adults.

Myth: Consuming too many food additives can cause ADHD.

Fact: There may be a subgroup of people with ADHD who are sensitive to certain food substances. But a recent study showed only 5 percent of people experienced a decrease in symptoms after consuming a special diet free of food additives.

Myth: Adult ADHD is a curse for life.

Fact: If properly treated, most adults with ADHD can live productive lives and learn to deal with their symptoms.

ADHD continues to be a disorder that is widely misunderstood by the general public, including many people who have the condition but never realize it. By knowing the myths, you can focus on symptoms that actually signal adult ADHD.

Diagnostic, Evaluation, and Treatment Basics

People with adult ADHD suffer from a galaxy of symptoms which can be organized under the categories of disorganization, impulsivity, restlessness, difficulty focusing attention, emotional instability, and low stress tolerance.

While some medical experts are able to make a diagnosis after simply talking with patients and observing their behavior, the vast majority of doctors rely on a combination of diagnostic techniques and evaluation tools to arrive at a definitive diagnosis. These may include interviews with patients, parents, teachers, friends, and colleagues; evaluating past and current school, college, and work records and performance reviews; and administering various tests that measure intelligence, aptitude, and other criteria.

The Challenges of Getting a Diagnosis

Because there is no single test to confirm a diagnosis of adult ADHD, making an assessment is often challenging and time-consuming. Getting an accurate diagnosis can be further complicated by the overlap between the symptoms of adult ADHD and those of other common psychiatric conditions such as depression and substance abuse.

In addition, most of the information about the etiology, symptoms, and treatment of the disorder still comes from observations of, and studies involving, children. Still another challenge is the tendency of some adults to diagnose themselves using unscientific online tests.

Alert

Don't assume you have adult ADHD until you see a medical specialist and get a diagnosis. According to research, nearly half of adults who self-diagnose don't have the condition, possibly because the disorder gets so much hype and exposure in the lay media.

Even if you meet diagnostic criteria, your family physician may be uncomfortable evaluating and treating an adult with symptoms of ADHD, particularly if you weren't diagnosed with childhood ADHD. Because the most effective treatment for the condition is the long-term use of stimulant drugs that have a high potential for abuse, some family physicians who aren't experts in treating the condition may be understandably reluctant to prescribe these drugs, and may prefer you consult with an adult ADHD specialist.

Evaluation Nuts and Bolts

Because an adult with ADHD may have considerable difficulty accurately recalling childhood behavior, his doctor may also ask him to provide any available school records and gather information from adults who knew him as a child. Physicians may also ask for job performance reviews that may indicate chronic inattentive, tardiness, distraction, and problems working with others.

Your physician may also want to talk to your spouse, close friends, and colleagues. She will also examine current and past therapies, ask about prescription and over-the-counter drug use, and inquire if you've ever used illegal drugs.

You may be asked to take simple tests to see if you have trouble with short-term memory loss and concentration. Your medical evaluation may also include a neurological examination. Laboratory tests may include a serum lead level and thyroid function tests, which can be used to rule out existing conditions, like thyroid disease, that share many symptoms with adult ADHD.

Treatment Overview

Although there is no proven "cure" for adult ADHD, the good news is you don't have to live with the symptoms. Medication frequently helps.

Approaches that attempt to modify brain function using biofeedback appear to help many people. You may also benefit from more traditional types of psychotherapy.

In addition, there is a world of complementary treatments at your disposal, including counseling, coaching, marriage and family therapy, and support groups. Although medication is often the first line of treatment, you may also need help with the practical aspects of your life, such as organizing, prioritizing, meeting deadlines, and accomplishing goals.

Strategies for Living

If you have adult ADHD, you know how difficult it can be to live and cope with the disorder. Many people may have trouble getting and keeping a job because they tend to change employers frequently or quit because they're bored. Because of poor job performance and problems relating to coworkers and supervisors, adults with ADHD are also fired more often than other workers.

When it comes to friendship and romances, many adults with ADHD have difficult personality traits that tend to drive people away. They also suffer a much higher rate of divorce, separation, and marital problems than other people.

Fact

According to research, problems with time management and other executive skills take a heavy toll on adults with ADHD. Twenty-five percent of them drop out of school, only 12 percent earn a bachelor's degree, and just 4 percent establish and maintain a professional career.

Although living with adult ADHD isn't easy, the good news is there are ever-increasing avenues of help, including life coaches, counselors, therapists, time management specialists, and others. Because the disease is so prevalent and so many adults are never diagnosed, more and more research is being conducted. Researchers are also developing better diagnostic tools so that fewer people slip through the cracks, and the search for more effective medications and treatments with fewer side effects has intensified.

Getting a Handle on Time

Many people with adult ADHD have a hard time determining how much they can really accomplish in a given time. Life or career coaches can help you learn not to bite off more than you can chew. They can also help you figure how much time you have in your schedule for a given task and plan accordingly. For instance, a coach can show you how to break big projects into smaller projects and assign a deadline for completing each part in order to catch problems before they snowball into major issues.

 Fact

Posting deadlines will help remind you to use your time wisely. Post them where you're likely to see them, such as on the refrigerator, microwave, or a wall near your desk, or create a computer screensaver. You can also put a note by your bed so it's the last thing you think about at night and the first thing you see when you wake up.

Successful Interpersonal Relationships

People with adult ADHD tend to fall into one of two categories. They may be loners, hermits, and extremely withdrawn and antisocial; or they may be so social that they can't stand being alone for an hour. Unfortunately, both extremes make it difficult for them to function in society.

Adults with ADHD often have a difficult time making and keeping meaningful relationships, whether it's with friends or marital partners. They tend to be impulsive and short-tempered and often drive people away. Because they may not have a clear sense of who they are or what they've done, it is often difficult for them to acknowledge and correct their offending behavior. Psychotherapy and biofeedback can help people recognize their negative personality traits, understand how their actions and comments affect others, and take steps to modify their behavior.

Like Parent, Like Child?

Researchers now know that ADHD is passed down from one generation to the next. If one parent has ADHD, there's a 40 percent chance that the child will inherit the condition. If both parents have ADHD, the child is 80 percent likely to inherit it. While the disorder is not behavioral in the sense that sufferers choose to behave in a certain way, the physiological characteristics of adult ADHD prompt those with the condition to respond to certain situations in certain ways.

Not a Life Sentence

Although ADHD is a highly genetic disorder, and it certainly presents myriad challenges to living a normal life, one of the most important things to remember is that it does not have to be a life sentence. Treatment can go a long way toward getting adult ADHD in check. Also, as you start to experience small successes in your newfound abilities to organize and prioritize your life or get along better with people, you may even begin to appreciate the silver lining of adult ADHD.

Having struggled with symptoms for years, you may find it difficult to believe that adult ADHD has a bright side. But the fact is that many artists, writers, producers, directors, scientists, inventors, physicists, mathematicians, and politicians throughout history have not only lived with the syndrome, but used their creativity and unique ability to think outside the box and attain great fame and fortune.

True, not everyone with adult ADHD has the IQ of Albert Einstein or the artistic genius of Steven Spielberg (both of whom dealt with the condition), but if you can imagine the world without the telephone, electricity, and rocket science, you can understand how different twenty-first century life would be without the many inventions, discoveries, and artistic masterpieces contributed by adults with ADHD.

CHAPTER 2

Understanding the Symptoms

C haracterized by inattention, hyperactivity, and impulsiveness, ADHD nearly always begins in childhood and often continues into adulthood. Researchers now believe that 60 percent of children with ADHD go on to have the disorder as adults. That translates into 4 percent of the adult population, or about 8 million adults. Unfortunately, for many reasons, only 15 percent of adults are ever diagnosed or treated. While learning to recognize the symptoms of ADHD may take time and effort, it can save you and your loved ones a lifetime of grief and unhappiness.

The Three Types of Adult ADHD

Scientists once believed that ADHD was mostly a problem with attention deficit. More recently, the disorder has been reclassified as a condition with three distinct subsets: inattentive, hyperactive-impulsive, and combination type. Although very few adults with ADHD fit neatly into one type of ADHD, they are diagnosed as having one type of the disorder over another when most of their symptoms seem to fall into that particular subset.

Most Common Types of Adult ADHD

By far the most common type of adult ADHD is the combination type, which affects up to 75 percent of all adult sufferers and is the major focus of this book. Inattentive ADHD, also called ADD, is the second most common type of adult ADHD and affects about 20 percent of adults with the condition. Hyperactive-impulsive ADHD is the least common subset in adults and affects only about 5 percent of people with adult ADHD.

ADHD symptoms such as hyperactivity and impulsiveness tend to appear before inattentiveness, and are highly prevalent in childhood ADHD. In adults, however, hyperactivity is usually the least predominant symptom while inattention is typically the most prevalent. This inattention wreaks havoc on the ability to perform a wide range of executive functions, including organizing, planning, prioritizing, setting goals, meeting deadlines, and breaking down large assignments into a series of smaller tasks.

Primary Symptoms

The primary symptoms of adult ADHD include impulsivity, inattention, and hyperactivity. They are called primary symptoms because they constitute the main indicators medical doctors look for when diagnosing the disorder. Each of the three symptoms has related problems.

The Problems with Impulsivity

If you're an adult with ADHD symptoms of impulsivity, you probably do a lot of things for emotional, rather than logical, reasons. Maybe you engage in impulse spending at the mall, or you choose tasks that offer immediate gratification and a short-term payoff while avoiding long-term projects that may not show results for months or years.

Although there are hundreds of different ways that impulsivity in adult ADHD can manifest itself, here are some common behaviors associated with impulsivity that you may recognize in yourself or in others with adult ADHD.

- You tend to blurt out inappropriate comments or put your foot in your mouth in social settings.
- You may constantly interrupt conversations or intrude without seeming to realize you're doing so.
- You often act without regard for future consequences; for instance, you engage in risky behavior like driving too fast or investing in risky financial schemes.
- You may have a short temper and struggle to contain your emotions. You may throw child-like temper tantrums at home when things don't go your way.
- You often display a lack of patience for societal niceties and regulations. For instance, you may refuse to wait in line at the grocery store or bank and butt in line, or you may decide you're in too much of a rush to wait and run a red light.

From Inattentive to Totally Zoned Out

If you suffer from inattention, you tend to zone out when the topic at hand isn't interesting or fascinating to you. You have a tendency to avoid, put off, or shirk tasks you consider mundane or boring. The flip side of being inattentive is being hyperattentive, or being so obsessed with one aspect of a task that not even repeated warnings from your boss can get you back on track.

Because you're usually operating at one extreme of inattention or the other, it seems you're always screwing up without understanding why. The following are some common ways that inattention can manifest itself in your life:

- You may be unable to stay focused on projects and tasks at work or at home.
- You often have trouble listening carefully when addressed directly by a boss, colleague, spouse, or significant other.

- You tend to have difficulty organizing and planning.
- You often can't be bothered with reading or following instructions or directions.
- You struggle to meet deadlines.
- You tend to misplace things you need to complete assignments and projects.
- You're likely to become bored, distracted, and withdrawn when you consider a subject or task boring or beneath you.
- You may routinely forget to do important things at home, such as taking out the garbage or picking up the mail.

Hyperactivity

If you have hyperactive symptoms, you're likely to be an on-the-go type who has trouble sitting still for long. You may be so impatient, wired, and restless that sitting through a meeting or even a movie is torture for you.

Fact

Only 50 percent of adults with ADHD are able to hold down full-time jobs, compared to 72 percent of adults without it. Studies also show that adults with ADHD earn $8,000 less per year than their peers. Research shows adults with ADHD in the United States suffer a collective $77 billion in lost earnings annually.

When it comes to your social life, you're likely to be a live wire in all the wrong ways. You may put your foot in your mouth often, jump into conversations or situations where you're not welcome, or wear out and exhaust your friends, colleagues, and family with your manic chatter or wacko, off-the-wall behavior.

The following are some other tell-tale signs that you may be suffering from hyperactivity symptoms of adult ADHD.

- You may need to be busy simply for the sake of being busy.
- You often talk incessantly and constantly interrupt people.
- You tend to drive way too fast for the road and weather conditions.
- You may have trouble slowing down enough to enjoy leisure activities like reading, sex, watching a movie, or getting a massage.
- You may have a number of nervous tics, such as tapping your feet, drumming your fingers, or tapping your pencil.
- When given a complicated assignment at work, you try to do everything at once instead of breaking it down into smaller pieces. You soon become so overwhelmed and panic-stricken that you shut down long before the project is completed.
- You abuse street drugs and alcohol to help yourself relax.
- You don't get much sleep.

Poor Executive Functioning

One of the biggest tell-tale signs of adult ADHD is a lack of "executive functioning," or the ability to redirect attention, inhibit inappropriate behavior, make decisions, switch problem-solving strategies, organize, prioritize, and get things done on time. Because executive functioning affects all areas of your life, especially your job, it can make getting and keeping a job an absolute nightmare. People with adult ADHD tend to disappoint and baffle their bosses and spouses, and this may isolate them even more.

Secondary Symptoms

In addition to primary symptoms, there are also many secondary symptoms of adult ADHD. Perhaps the most significant symptom is the tendency to be disorganized, a trait shared by people who suffer from all three types of the disorder. An inability to organize can turn simple tasks like keeping track of records and paperwork into a nightmare both for adults with ADHD and the people who live and work with them.

Adults with ADHD also have an inability to plan ahead. They tend to live from crisis to crisis, which provides the stimulation and excitement they may crave, but ultimately backfires on them when bosses, friends, and spouses get fed up. Because of their impulsiveness and hyperactivity, adults with ADHD also have a tendency to change horses midstream, either because of boredom or because the planning and details involved seem insurmountable.

The Two Sides of Adult ADHD

The good news is adult ADHD isn't all bad. In fact, many researchers attribute adult ADHD's unique brain wiring to an ability to think outside the box, solve complex mathematical puzzles, and invent new forms of art, music, and films. From presidents and inventors to artists and musicians, many famous people with adult ADHD succeeded beyond their wildest dreams. For now, here are some of the more common positive attributes shared by adults with ADHD.

The Positive Side

Adults with ADHD tend to rely on their gut feelings. This may also explain why so many counselors, psychologists, psychiatrists, pastors, and priests have adult ADHD.

Many people with adult ADHD are very creative in the way they tackle problems and find solutions. They are also creative by nature; many writers, artists, and filmmakers, including a number of celebrities, have adult ADHD.

Adults with ADHD also tend to be very intelligent, even if they don't always score well on IQ tests. The problem is that adults with the disorder become bored very easily. If that online IQ test isn't absolutely captivating or fascinating, you're likely to turn off your computer.

The Negative Side

As an adult with ADHD, you're also likely to display some negative character traits that can make it difficult for you to get along with people.

You may feel that other people just don't "get" you—and you may be right! The fact is that many people don't really understand adult ADHD and some are skeptical that it is an actual condition.

As an adult with ADHD, you may also think and process information differently than other people because of the inherent differences in the way your brain is wired. This can leave you open to ridicule and criticism, which may make you feel like an oddball or outcast.

Essential

People with adult ADHD have trouble finishing things because they tend to be overly obsessive and perfectionist in their thinking. In fact, many adults with ADHD believe there is no such thing as a finished product. They may also become too overwhelmed with a project to continue and give up long before it's due.

Trouble getting and staying organized is another major trait of adults with ADHD. You may also be so disorganized that you rarely get things done on time, fail to do the most important things first, or forget when things are due. Time may seem like a foreign concept to you, and you may often appear to be in your own time zone, oblivious to the deadlines that affect the rest of the world.

If you're an adult with ADHD who fails to complete work projects, pay bills on time, or remember important dates, not getting the job done is only one consequence of your inaction. You may also come across as extremely arrogant, self-centered, and narcissistic, as well as oblivious to the needs and desires of anyone but yourself.

The Silver Lining of Adult ADHD

Since thinking outside the box is one of your many fortes you can, by using a little positive thinking, reframe all those negative traits into positive traits that actually work in your favor. For instance, if you're feeling inattentive, it could be a sign that you're just not cut out for that type of work and that you need to keep looking until you find a good fit for your gifts and talents.

Your natural impulsivity may be a drawback when you hit the mall or a Vegas casino, but it can also help you make a leap of faith or take a courageous stand that others might find daunting. It also means you're not likely to stay in a bad situation for long.

There's no doubt that having a high energy level, or being hyperactive, can make it tough to sit still through a long meeting. But it can also be a real asset when you need to get something done, especially since your tendency to hyperfocus means you'll probably devote your full attention to it.

In short, having adult ADHD doesn't have to be a curse. While it poses many challenges, you may have some special gifts and talents that friends and colleagues without the disorder can only dream of.

Other Problems Associated with Adult ADHD

Adults with ADHD also suffer from a host of miscellaneous problems regarding interpersonal relationships and their ability to cope at work and at home. In fact, the classic symptoms of adult ADHD can unravel marriages and friendships.

Studies show that adults with ADHD have a higher rate of marital problems and multiple marriages than the general public, and they also have a higher incidence of separation and divorce. If children are involved, the stakes are even higher.

Trouble at Work

Getting and keeping a job in a challenging job market presents special challenges to adults with ADHD, who must compete with more and more people for fewer and fewer jobs. You must not only have the necessary training, talent, and experience, but you must also be adept at planning, organizing, prioritizing, paying attention to detail, and focusing on important things—areas in which many adults with ADHD have difficulties.

Because of your natural impulsiveness and hyperactivity, you may be more likely to quit a job when the going gets tough and seek out greener pastures in the form of a job with less responsibility, less stress, and fewer hassles. Unfortunately, such jobs may also provide less income.

Conditions That Overlap or Mimic Adult ADHD

Many psychiatric conditions—including anxiety, depression, substance abuse, and personality disorders—mimic or mask the symptoms of adult ADHD. Sometimes it's hard for a medical expert to know which disease or condition is causing which symptoms and how to best treat them.

A high percentage of adults with ADHD also suffer from comorbid disorders that commonly occur alongside adult ADHD, and which may exacerbate a physician's attempt to isolate and treat symptoms. The most common overlapping diseases and conditions include clinical depression and anxiety, bipolar disorder, substance abuse, alcoholism, learning disorders, dyslexia, fibromyalgia, brain injuries, dementia, psychosis, hypothyroidism, hyperthyroidism, conduct disorder, speech and communication problems, sensory integration disorders, oppositional defiance disorder, and sleep disorders.

People with untreated thyroid conditions, including hypothyroidism and hyperthyroidism, often display symptoms presented in adult ADHD. Individuals who are hypothyroid (the thyroid is too slow) are often depressed, lethargic, and disinterested, while those who are hyperthyroid (the thyroid is too fast) tend to be irritable, nervous, anxious, agitated, and excitable.

Research also shows that adults with ADHD are affected by many other problems, including erratic moods, rollercoaster emotions, a short temper, chronic pessimism, a constant craving for stimulation, a desire not to be touched, highly fluctuating energy levels, clumsiness, and problems with hand-eye coordination. Psychotics are sometimes able to convince friends, family, and even their medical doctors that their real problem is undiagnosed and untreated adult ADHD.

Medications and Drugs That May Mask Symptoms

Although you normally think of medication as something that heals or cures a condition, when it comes to adult ADHD some medications produce symptoms that actually mimic the disorder. For instance, that flu medicine you took this morning may have left you feeling nervous, jittery, and irritable, while the sleeping pill you took the night before may have left you feeling confused and lethargic. Whether it's a seemingly benign over-the-counter pill for a headache, a prescription drug your doctor ordered, or an illegal drug you took because you thought it might help you relax, nearly every drug has side effects that can affect you.

 Alert

Studies show that adults with ADHD are twice as likely to smoke as people who don't have the disorder, and are also more inclined to be heavy coffee drinkers. In addition, they are also at a much higher risk for abusing illegal drugs, prescription drugs, and alcohol.

If you think you may have adult ADHD, your doctor will probably ask you to stop taking your medications until he can figure out which symptoms are caused by the medication and which symptoms are caused by the disorder. If you are already addicted to one or more illegal drugs, your doctor may recommend that you undergo detoxification or enter a rehab program before starting treatment for adult ADHD.

Over-the-Counter Drugs

Allergy medications like Claritin and Zyrtec can cause restlessness, nervousness, sleeplessness, excitability, and poor coordination. Diet pills may contain excessive amounts of stimulants like caffeine or green tea that result in nervousness, anxiety, restlessness, an inability to focus, and insomnia. Sleeping pills can cause confusion, lethargy, and apathy. Cold and flu tablets and syrups that contain antihistamine-decongestant combinations like pseudoephedrine and/or phenylephrine can cause excitability, nervousness, anxiety, and sleeplessness.

Over-the-counter drugs are easy to abuse because they don't require a prescription. To ensure your doctor doesn't confuse the side effects of over-the-counter medications with symptoms of adult ADHD, write down a list of everything you take, including dosage details.

Prescription Drugs

Many prescription drugs also have side effects that can mimic symptoms of adult ADHD. Here is a list of some prescription drugs whose side effects may be mistaken for adult ADHD symptoms.

- Beta blockers: Common side effects include confusion, depression, and memory loss.
- Wellbutrin, prescribed for depression and anxiety as well as smoking cessation: Side effects include nervousness, lightheadedness, excitability, insomnia, nightmares, difficulty concentrating, anger and hostility, depression, and loss of interest.

- Anticonvulsants like Klonopin: Common side effects include poor muscle control and behavioral changes.
- Oral contraceptives: Side effects include depression, nervousness, and tiredness and fatigue.
- Benzodiazepam tranquilizers like Valium and Ativan: Side effects include confusion, depression, lethargy, nervousness, hysteria, and tremors.
- Selective serotonin reuptake inhibitors (SSRIs) prescribed for depression: Common side effects include anxiety, nervousness, sleeplessness, and changes in sex drive.
- Thyroid replacement drugs: Common side effects include nervousness, anxiety, sleeplessness, and heart palpitations.

As with over-the-counter drugs, make a list and give it to your medical doctor so he doesn't confuse side effects for symptoms that may indicate adult ADHD.

Substance Abuse

Unfortunately, many adults with undiagnosed adult ADHD use illegal drugs to mask the symptoms of their disorder. In fact, studies show adult ADHD is associated with an earlier onset of substance abuse, a longer period of active abuse, and a lower rate of recovery. Adults with ADHD may use a variety of illegal drugs to mask social phobias, nervousness, anxiety, insomnia, an inability to concentrate and focus, and other tell-tale signs of adult ADHD. These drugs include cocaine, marijuana, street amphetamines, street tranquilizers, and the illegal use of stimulant prescription drugs like Ritalin, Adderall, and Concertal.

By the time a patient sees a doctor for adult ADHD, he may already be addicted to a drug that requires a detoxification program. Although stimulant medications like Ritalin and Adderall are commonly prescribed for adult ADHD, they should never be taken without a doctor's supervision or used for off-label purposes like weight loss.

CHAPTER 3

Searching for Causes

S cientists still don't know exactly what causes adult ADHD or what conditions are responsible for the disorder. Most agree that ADHD is a neurological disorder of the nervous system that affects several areas of the brain, including those responsible for behavior, working memory, and executive functions. Researchers also know that adult ADHD is a highly genetic disease. Unfortunately, the symptoms of adult ADHD manifest differently in different people, so it can be difficult to recognize and diagnose.

Five Current Theories

One of the first questions you may ask after you've been diagnosed with adult ADHD is, "Did I do something wrong to cause it?" Over the years, medical science has come up with many theories regarding what might cause ADHD. Today, most researchers agree that the disorder is not only highly genetic, but that it also has a neurobiological cause.

Here are five current theories as to what may cause ADHD.

1. ADHD is caused by structural abnormalities in the brain. Research using magnetic resonance imagers (MRIs) has shown that four brain regions in children with ADHD are smaller than those in children without ADHD.

2. ADHD is caused by an insufficient supply of the neurotransmitter dopamine in the brain. This theory would explain why stimulant medications that increase dopamine in the brain are effective in controlling ADHD symptoms. Researchers speculate that the lack of dopamine may affect how it interacts with two other neurotransmitters, norepinephrine and serotonin.

3. ADHD is really a sleep disorder in disguise. Some researchers believe the disorder may be caused by a sleep-deprived brain, and the hyperactivity people with ADHD exhibit may be an effort to compensate for drowsiness. Many people with ADHD have sleep disorders, while others sleep so soundly it's hard to wake them up.

4. ADHD is a hereditary condition. While researchers don't fully understand why and how ADHD is passed from one generation to the next, they agree there is a strong genetic component. Children with ADHD are extremely likely to have at least one close relative with the disorder.

5. Environmental agents such as cigarette and alcohol use during pregnancy may increase the risk of ADHD in children. High levels of lead may also cause ADHD.

Ten Theories That Have Been Debunked

Although most experts have largely discounted earlier theories about the causes of ADHD, some of them continue to persist.

1. Food additives and sugar cause ADHD. A study conducted in 1982 by the NIH found that restricting sugar in the diets of children with ADHD was beneficial in just 5 percent of cases, mostly in children who already had food allergies. There is no research indicating that excess sugar consumption causes ADHD, although it may cause hyperactivity in some people.

2. The dramatic rise of ADHD in recent years is caused by increased toxins in the environment. While it's true that both the incidence of ADHD in children and adults and the amount of toxins in the environment has increased, there are no studies indicating a link between the two. In fact, experts largely attribute the increase in ADHD to advances in diagnostic tools.

3. Exposure to lead causes ADHD. The accumulation of lead in the brain was once believed to cause ADHD. While research has shown that some people with ADHD may not tolerate lead as well as people who don't have the disorder, there is no definite research linking lead to ADHD.

4. ADHD is caused by brain damage. This early theory originated around the time of the 1918 flu epidemic, when affected children came down with symptoms that resembled ADHD, including hyperactivity, inattentiveness, and impulsivity. This theory was later refuted, but it nevertheless paved the way for the state-of-the-art research that is being conducted today.

5. ADHD is caused by traumatic brain injury resulting from a lack of oxygen during birth or from a head injury in early childhood. That brain injuries have many symptoms that overlap or mimic the symptoms of ADHD led researchers to suspect a correlation between the two. No studies have confirmed this theory.

6. Allergies and food sensitivities trigger ADHD. While these conditions have symptoms that may mimic or overlap with the symptoms of ADHD, there is no research showing a connection between the two. Most people see a dramatic reduction or elimination of their food allergy symptoms when they begin medication for the condition.

7. A poor diet causes ADHD. While malnutrition has not been linked with ADHD, some studies show that a lack of omega-3 fatty acids in the diet may exacerbate ADHD symptoms.

These fats are important for brain development and function, and having insufficient amounts may contribute to, if not actually cause, developmental disorders in children. Fish oil supplements appear to decrease the symptoms of ADHD in some children and adults and may even help them improve their performance at school and at work.

8. ADHD is the result of "moral defectiveness." This early theory claimed that people with ADHD were morally defective by nature. While many people with ADHD suffer from behavioral issues that lead to problems later in life, there is no evidence the disorder is caused by an inherent moral defectiveness.

9. ADHD is a willful behavior caused by defiance. This theory puts the blame on parents, claiming that children who fail to pay attention could be "cured" if parents taught them not to misbehave or daydream. It assumes that children with ADHD were being inattentive, impulsive, and defiant by choice. Unfortunately, many people today continue to believe that ADHD is a fictional disease used to excuse everything from lax parenting to misbehavior.

10. ADHD is caused by a poor upbringing. This early theory remains one of the leading misconceptions about ADHD today. While improper parenting can exacerbate the symptoms of ADHD, research shows that being overly strict with children and teenagers who suffer from the disorder nearly always backfires. Studies show that while ADHD symptoms can't be scolded or disciplined away, a variety of treatment modalities, including medication, psychotherapy, and biofeedback, can help decrease or even eliminate them.

Research Overview

ADHD has had many different names since the early 1900s, many of which reflected the current thinking of the time. Before the disorder was officially recognized by the American Psychiatric Association (APA) as a mental disorder in the mid-1980s, ADHD was called Minimal Brain Damage and Minimal Brain Dysfunction. Since then, the disorder has been renamed many times in the APA's *Diagnostic and Statistic Manual of Mental Disorders (DSM)*. The first edition of the *DSM* called it "hyperactivity of childhood." The second edition, published in 1968, changed the name to "hyperkinetic reaction of children." In 1980, the third edition of the *DSM* renamed it "attention deficit disorder with or without hyperactivity."

Fact

Don't get too attached to the name ADHD. Ongoing studies indicate that symptoms may arise in various places in the brain. If this proves to be true, ADHD could one day be divided into five to seven different disorders, each with its own symptoms and treatments. Or the disorder could remain ADHD, but be reclassified as having five to seven subsets, rather than the three it has today.

The abbreviation ADD is still used interchangeably with ADHD outside the medical community, but technically the name has changed. In 1988, a text revision of the third edition of the *DSM* revised the name to "attention deficit hyperactivity disorder, or ADHD." In 1994, the fourth edition of the *DSM* added a slash, and revised the name to AD/HD. Although the name of the disorder may undergo more changes in the future as research evolves, for now, the most popular term for the disorder is ADHD.

So What's Taking So Long?

Given the dramatic advances in technology, you may be wondering how and why scientists could figure out how to send a man to the moon, but still not understand what causes a biological disorder that affects millions of people.

The easiest response is that the human brain is a complicated labyrinth. Scientists now know that the primary symptom of adult ADHD is an inability to self-regulate, or to control attention, temper, moods, and impulses.

Fact

The NIH conducted a landmark study in 1990 that showed there was reduced glucose uptake in the brains of ADHD adults compared with "normal" people. This study established a biological basis for ADHD by providing a measurable difference between the ADHD and non-ADHD brain. But scientists still don't understand where the difference comes from or exactly what it means.

Everything you do is partly the result of your unique brain wiring and partly the result of learned experiences. As an adult with ADHD, you may not be able to fully integrate learned experiences and, as a result, you may be developmentally younger than your peers and may perform at lower levels.

Your Brain and Executive Function

Several areas of your brain are responsible for controlling executive functions, or brain functions you need to control and regulate your behavior. Some scientists believe the root cause of ADHD lies with response inhibition, or the ability to control your impulses, stay focused, and delay immediate gratification. They also believe this core problem negatively impacts the brain's many other executive functions.

Other executive functions affected by a lack of response inhibition are motor control, which includes hand-eye coordination and the ability to control impulsive movements like finger or foot tapping; regulating your emotions; motivation; and planning. With advances in technology, scientists are now able to explore the brain for abnormalities that could result in ADHD. While past research focused almost exclusively on external factors like parental upbringing, environmental causes, and toxic culprits like sugar and lead, research today targets genetic, anatomical, functional, and chemical brain dysfunctions as potential causes of the disorder.

Your Memory and Adult ADHD

Memory is a highly complex process scattered across many parts of your brain. Simply put, your memory is a system of taking in or acquiring information; coding, filing, and storing it; and retrieving it as you need it.

Adults with ADHD don't necessarily have a bad memory so much as a defect in one or more links of the highly complex chain that makes up memory. By understanding how this process works, you can improve or simply bypass those broken links.

Breaks in the Acquisition Chain

For some adults with ADHD, the broken links occur in the process of acquiring memory. How much you acquire is related to your interest or need for the information, your motivation to acquire it, and your ability to process the information. People with ADHD have considerable trouble remembering details that don't seem important, interesting, or relevant. They may tune out information when they aren't motivated to remember it, or when the information seems boring or repetitive. Many adults with ADHD also lack the patience and focus to sort, process, code, and file information so it's easier to retrieve when they need it later.

Breaks in the Storage Chain

For other people with ADHD, the problem is with storing memory. Many adults with ADHD have defective filters, meaning they have trouble screening out unnecessary data. Instead of sorting the necessary data from the unnecessary, they take it all in. The result is information overload, which can short-circuit working memory. Short-term memory, another type of temporary storage, is also highly vulnerable to distraction and lack of focus, both of which are major challenges for adults with ADHD.

Long-term memory is your vault of safe-deposit boxes in which you code and store facts, experiences, knowledge, values, and routines. When you go grocery shopping and see an apple, orange, and banana, your long-term memory retrieves them from a safe-deposit box you've already labeled "fruits." With knowledge and experience, you cross-reference each fruit to other fruits by association and create even more coded safe-deposit boxes. For instance, "orange" may be filed in a "citrus" safe-deposit box along with grapefruit and lemon and in another safe-deposit box labeled "fruit that grows on trees" along with apples and pears.

Most adults with ADHD are excellent at thinking outside the box, and they also tend to have active imaginations. While creating an endless succession of different safe-deposit boxes for "orange" poses no problem for them, they might be so prone to distraction that they leave an entire grocery cart of fruit sitting in the parking lot.

Breaks in the Access Stage

When you access information from your memory, you either recognize it as familiar or you retrieve information using specific recall. The ability to recall precise information relies on the way you've stored the information. If you've rote-memorized information with no thought to associating or cross-referencing it to other stored information, you may have trouble remembering it because it's not important. Many adults with adult ADHD are so averse to details, organizing, and planning that their memory files are haphazard.

Breaks in Transfer

Transfer is a complex memory process in which you reshuffle pieces of data to form new knowledge. It can include finding a commonality between divergent ideas or combining unrelated pieces of information into a whole new idea. Many adults with

ADHD, being highly creative thinkers, excel at combining wildly divergent ideas into new and creative songs, plots, and works of art. They can also combine their knowledge to solve problems in ways that would never occur to people with more orderly or logical minds. It's no surprise that many famous producers, artists, musicians, physicists, mathematicians, and inventors had adult ADHD.

Searching for Causes

There's much disagreement when it comes to the causes of ADHD, but many scientists agree that ADHD has a strong genetic basis in the majority of cases. In fact, the first thing your physician may ask if he suspects you have adult ADHD is if anyone else in your family has it.

Searching for ADHD Genes

Genetic researchers now believe ADHD is actually an umbrella term for several slightly different disorders. Because ADHD is one of the most heritable of psychiatric disorders, researchers have been searching for genes that underlie the disorder in the hopes that gene discovery will lead to better treatments.

Fact

Research from all over the world is being collected and published by the ADHD Molecular Genetics Network. While scientists have been able to identify some genes that may be associated with ADHD, it still isn't clear what causes those genes to become defective.

The largest genetic study of ADHD was recently conducted at the International ADHD Multicenter Genetics (IMAGE) project at the State University of New York (SUNY) Upstate Medical Center. The studies examined more than 600,000 genetic markers in more than 900 families and found one genetic marker that may be associated with ADHD symptoms. Studies also suggest that genes are involved in ADHD and that each of these have small effects, although larger studies are needed to confirm the initial findings and fully understand the genetic mechanisms underlying ADHD.

Another study at SUNY examined genetic markers across the entire human genome to search for genes that may someday be used to predict which people will respond most favorably to stimulant medications used to treat ADHD.

The research indicated that while genetic factors may impact the effectiveness of stimulants in alleviating ADHD symptoms, no single gene appears to have a substantial impact on treatment response.

The Genetic Connection

A wide range of studies on twins, adopted children, and specific genes associated with ADHD have explored how and why ADHD is passed on from one generation to the next. This research has provided enlightening clues that may help scientists unravel the mysteries of ADHD.

Research conducted at the University of Massachusetts showed that parents or siblings of someone with ADHD are 30 to 80 percent more likely to have ADHD than someone who doesn't have close relatives with the disorder. At the University of California, research indicated that ADHD traits such as hostility, aggression, and a constant craving for excitement and thrills may, in fact, be caused by two specific inherited genes. Studies conducted on twins by scientists at the University of South Wales in Australia concluded that if one twin had ADHD, the other twin was 81 percent likely to have it as well.

Environment versus Genetics

Research has also followed the impact of hereditary versus environmental factors on adopted children with ADHD raised by nonbiological parents. One study concluded that genes had more influence on childhood ADHD than upbringing or environment. Another study showed that adopted children had a more than 30 percent chance of having ADHD. While this contradicts claims that genetics overrides environment when it comes to ADHD, it fits in well with psychodynamic theories claiming the trauma of early separation from biological parents can result in hyperactivity and behavioral problems.

 Fact

In families where one parent and one child already have ADHD, every successive child born to that parent has the same chance of getting ADHD as the first child—a 30 to 80 percent chance of being born with the disorder.

A Rare Thyroid Disorder Provides Clues

The NIH discovered a startling association between ADHD and a rare genetic thyroid disorder. The condition, called generalized resistance to thyroid hormone, occurs in just one in 100,000 people, or about 50 families in the United States. People with the disorder are resistant to the action of the thyroid hormone, which regulates a host of important functions in the body, including metabolism, bone growth, and brain development.

Families with generalized resistance to thyroid hormone have a 50 to 70 percent chance of passing it on. Scientists still aren't sure whether ADHD occurs because the thyroid problem gets in the way of normal brain development, or if the thyroid condition and ADHD have a defective gene in common. Although this disease is extremely rare, researchers believe it may one day help shed light on what causes ADHD.

Exploring Brain Anatomy

With the advent of brain imaging technology such as MRI, positron emission tomography (PET) scans, and single proton emission computed tomography (SPECT) scans, scientists no longer have to guess what's going on in your brain. While they can't see your actual thought process, they are able to measure the size, shape, and symmetry of your brain and compare it against the brains of people who don't have ADHD.

However, researchers still don't know what causes "bad connections" in the brains of ADHD people. Is it caused by a smaller-sized brain or one that's not quite symmetrical? Do connections somehow misfire and get lost? Or is it a problem with our neurotransmitters, our brain's miniscule messengers?

Despite the dramatic increase in research, many answers continue to elude scientists, although they have made one major discovery. Using MRIs to scan the brains of people with ADHD, researchers have discovered that four regions in their brains are smaller than in "normal" brains.

A Look Inside Your Brain

Those four regions of the brain include the frontal lobes, the corpus collosum, the basal ganglia, and the cerebellum.

The frontal lobes are critical for executive functions like planning and organizing. Researchers already know that damage to the frontal lobes resulting from injury can result in mood swings, impulsivity, lack of inhibition, and hyperactivity.

The corpus collosum is the rope of nerves that connects the two hemispheres of your brain. Studies have shown that this area of the brain, besides being smaller in people with ADHD, also operates differently than in those who don't have the disorder.

The basal ganglia is a set of nuclei deep within your brain that connects the left and right frontal lobes and lets them talk to each other. Research has shown that basal ganglia that are asymmetrical or smaller in size may indicate a higher incidence of ADHD.

The cerebellum is the part of the brain responsible for balance and motor coordination. Having a smaller cerebellum than normal could explain why some people with undiagnosed ADHD have problems with hand-eye coordination.

The Role of Brain Function

ADHD brains not only look different from normal brains, they also function differently. Scientists can now compare the functioning of ADHD brains and "normal" brains.

One study used brain scans on adults with and without ADHD to measure the level of brain activity in their frontal lobes when they were concentrating, and again when they were at rest. The differences were startling.

When people with ADHD concentrated, the activity level in the frontal lobe decreased from its level at rest. In people without ADHD, just the opposite was true. This was a giant stepping stone in establishing ADHD as a biological disease.

ADHD and Brain Waves

At New York University, researchers found that subjects with ADHD showed eleven different patterns of brain waves when compared with the brain waves of "normal" people. Studies conducted at the University of Tennessee reported that people with ADHD showed an increase in slower brain waves in the frontal lobe region when they concentrated. This finding corresponds with other studies indicating a lower level of brain waves in this region.

Are Chemical Deficiencies the Culprit?

The brain and central nervous system work like a command center to coordinate every system in the human body. Comprised of millions of nerve cells, the command center receives and transmits signals from one part of the body to another.

Impulses are carried along the length of nerve cells and "jump" from one cell to another. The gap between nerve cells is called a synapse. The chemical messengers that carry the impulse across the gap are called neurotransmitters.

Meet Your Neurotransmitters

Epinephrine and norepinephrine are two neurotransmitters that mobilize the body's reaction to danger and trigger the "fight or flight" response you've probably experienced as a racing heart and heightened senses. Dopamine is a neurotransmitter that helps regulate your general activity level, whether you're active or passive, alert or disinterested, or awake or asleep.

Studies on Neurotransmitters

Many studies have shown a link between ADHD and an imbalance of neurotransmitters in the brain. Stimulant drugs used to treat ADHD relieve symptoms by increasing dopamine levels in the brain. Using indirect drug response research, researchers have discovered that insufficient levels of dopamine may be associated with ADHD.

Other studies associated ADHD with an imbalance of norepinephrine and dopamine in the brain. Having too much norepinephrine could make you feel agitated and in a constant state of fight or flight, a common symptom in adults with ADHD. Although scientists haven't yet pinpointed the exact mechanism that causes ADHD, they have discounted many older theories and are conducting promising research that suggests the disorder is caused by an imbalance of neurotransmitters in the brain.

If the condition proves to be not one but several different disorders, researchers may be able to isolate specific causes and treat them separately. The good news is that if you have adult ADHD, medical science is closer than ever to discovering the root causes behind it.

CHAPTER 4

The Many Faces of Adult ADHD

A DHD is a neurobiological disorder that affects people of every age, race, socioeconomic background, and culture. ADHD has long been viewed as a condition that primarily affects boys and men—and it does affect about twice as many men as women. However, that still means there are millions of women with the condition. Until the 1970s, researchers believed that ADHD was a childhood disease that children outgrew by puberty. Today, studies show that up to 50 percent of children with ADHD still have symptoms as adults.

Why Is Adult ADHD So Often Under-diagnosed?

Adult ADHD remains difficult to diagnose, especially in adults who were never diagnosed as children.

Absence of Childhood Diagnosis

As an adult, you can't be diagnosed with ADHD unless you've had the disorder since you were a child. This can be a stumbling block if you've suspected for years that you have the disorder, but were never diagnosed and may not have access to medical documentation detailing your behavior as a child.

Also, trying to recall specific symptoms from childhood can be daunting. Sometimes, enlisting the help of parents, teachers, and childhood friends can help a medical specialist fill in the missing pieces.

Right Symptoms, Wrong Disease

You already know that adult ADHD mimics the symptoms of many other mental disorders. In addition, some medical conditions, including thyroid disease and head injuries, have symptoms that may look like adult ADHD.

Ruling Out Overlapping Conditions

Many adults who have ADHD also have clinical depression, anxiety, bipolar disorder, and problems with substance abuse.

Adult ADHD versus Lifestyle Stress

Let your doctor know if you're going through a hellish life situation so he won't mistake normal reactions for the symptoms of adult ADHD.

Increased Role of Family Physicians

According to a study conducted at the New York University School of Medicine, 50 percent of family physicians don't feel confident diagnosing adult ADHD. In contrast, 2–3 percent feel comfortable diagnosing depression and anxiety disorders. A whopping 85 percent of family physicians surveyed said they would be more likely to diagnose and treat adult ADHD if they had a reliable, easy-to-use screening tool. Based on the results of the study, the World Health Organization (WHO) developed an ADHD screening test that patients can take at home.

The free online self-assessment test is available at *http://psych .med.nyu.edu/patient-care/adult-adhd-screening-test*. The results of this test do not constitute a diagnosis of adult ADHD, but they may provide the impetus for you to seek treatment.

Does Adult ADHD Always Begin in Childhood?

The answer is yes—always. Although the disorder is called adult ADHD when it affects adults, the adult version is actually an extension of childhood ADHD. There is no ADHD that begins in adulthood or that only affects adults.

However, this is not to suggest that the childhood and adult versions of ADHD are identical. ADHD is a neurobiological disorder that changes as you age, so the symptoms you experienced as a child are likely to be much different than those you experience as an adult.

In general, symptoms of hyperactivity decrease as you get older and symptoms of inattention, impulsivity, and problems with executive functions (planning, organizing, and prioritizing) tend to increase.

 Alert

Researchers believe that future studies on the developing brains of infants and young children may yield important clues as to what causes the onset of ADHD and why some brains never reach full maturity.

ADHD symptoms also manifest themselves in different ways as you age. Your symptoms of impulsiveness at ages seven and at age fifteen may bear little resemblance to the symptoms of impulsiveness as a forty-two-year-old.

Do All Children Have ADHD as Adults?

The answer is no. According to research conducted by the NIH, 50 percent of children with ADHD grow out of the disorder in their twenties. This is because certain brain regions in children with ADHD tend to mature later than normal.

The research used MRIs to compare the brains of 400 children with and without ADHD. The middle portion of the brain, responsible for controlling action and attention, matured later than normal in children with ADHD.

The study concluded that many children with ADHD eventually catch up with children without the disorder and experience a decrease in symptoms such as hyperactivity and inattention as they mature.

When Adult ADHD Affects Adult Teenagers

Dealing with raging hormones, peer pressure, and sexuality is hard enough. Add in undiagnosed ADHD and a teen's transition years from childhood to adulthood can be a trying time for everyone involved.

Numbers Tell the Story

Research shows that teenagers with undiagnosed ADHD may be walking time bombs on a variety of levels. Compared to "normal" teenagers (if such a thing exists), teenagers with ADHD are twice as likely to run away from home, three times as likely to be arrested, ten times as likely to get pregnant, and 400 times as likely to contract a sexually transmitted disease. Teenagers with impulsive ADHD are also a hazard behind the wheel, having a 400 percent greater risk of being in traffic accidents and receiving speeding tickets than other teens.

Studies estimate that up to 50 percent of teenagers in juvenile centers may suffer from undiagnosed Adult ADHD.

What Teenager ADHD Looks Like

Depression is common among teenagers, and some studies estimate that up to 25 percent of teenagers suffer from the condition. But unlike the gloom-and-doom strain of depression exhibited by adults, teenagers manifest their depression in different ways. They may belittle themselves, withdraw from society, feel rejected, or hang out with a bad crowd. Teenagers with adult ADHD are also far more likely than normal teenagers to engage in self-destructive behavior such as drug and alcohol abuse, sexual promiscuity, reckless driving, and dropping out of school.

ADHD Teenagers at School

The three major symptoms of ADHD—hyperactivity, impulsiveness, and inattention—wreak havoc on a teenager's ability to function at school. Many have difficulty sitting still, listening, and staying focused. They also experience problems with executive functions like taking and organizing notes, comprehending reading and homework assignments, and getting to class on time. They may also fail to turn in homework assignments or complete projects by the deadline.

Essential

Research conducted by the National Institute of Mental Health (NIMH) shows the teenage brain is a work in progress. Brain scans showed the structural changes in the brain that occur during late adolescence paralleled a pruning process that occurs early in life. It seems to follow a use-it-or-lose-it principle: neural connections that get exercised are retained, while those that don't are lost.

Many teenagers with ADHD are ostracized by classmates because of their impulsive or rude behavior. To get attention, boys may adopt sarcastic or smart aleck behavior while girls may resort to sexual promiscuity.

The Difference in Teenage Emotions

New research conducted at Harvard University confirms that teenagers process emotions differently than adults. MRIs were used to scan the brains of teenagers as they identified the emotions displayed by faces shown on computer screens. In young teenagers who performed poorly on the task, the amygdala—a brain center that mediates fear and other gut reactions—was activated more than the frontal lobe. As teenagers in the study got older, their brain activity shifted to the frontal lobe, resulting in more reasoned perceptions. The researchers also noted a similar shift in activation during language skills tasks in teenagers in the study.

College Students Coping with Adult ADHD

Every college or university with federal funding is obligated to provide "reasonable accommodations" for the estimated 2–4 percent of college students who have adult ADHD, but the amount of help varies widely among schools. Some schools provide the bare minimum to comply with the federal law. Others offer every imaginable service to accommodate students with adult ADHD, including student disability services, study skills programs, specialized help during registration and freshman orientation, on-campus physicians who specialize in treating ADHD, and access to on-campus ADHD coaches, counseling, psychotherapy, and support groups.

 Alert

College students with ADHD have more academic difficulties, fewer academic coping strategies, more intrusive thoughts, a higher degree of restlessness, and a lower quality of life than college students without ADHD, according to research presented at the August 2004 annual meeting of Children and Adults with ADHD (CHADD).

If you have adult ADHD, look for a college or university that has a welcoming and supportive attitude toward students with the disorder. The college you choose should go out of its way to facilitate the transition to college life. Work with your high school guidance counselor to hone in on colleges that have small class sizes, low student-to-professor ratios, and an emphasis on personalized attention.

To Disclose or Not to Disclose

There's no law saying you must disclose you have adult ADHD, but it may be the best choice for many people with adult ADHD. By disclosing your disability, you'll provide the admissions department with the information they need to make an informed decision about how well you're likely to fit in at their school. You may also be eligible for valuable assistance through the college's disabilities office.

Essential

College students diagnosed with ADHD may be eligible for services under Section 504 of the Rehabilitation Act of 1973 and the Americans with Disabilities Act. If you decide to disclose that you have adult ADHD, you will be required to submit documentation of your disorder. This may include records of psychological evaluations, the date of diagnosis, high school records that document special assistance you received, and a current IEP/504 plan.

Once you've decided on a college, register for disabilities services right away. To ensure you'll get the services you need from the start, apply for admissions and disabilities services at the same time.

College students with ADHD may qualify for the use of assistive technology to help them cope with their disability. These include voice-activated software, books on tape, personal organizers, and computer outlining programs.

Special Challenges for Students with Adult ADHD

In college, most of your life revolves around being able to concentrate, focus, retain knowledge, take good notes, schedule time for studying, and manage your time so that you get things done on time. Therefore, problems with executive functions can present a unique challenge.

Many students with ADHD overestimate what they can realistically accomplish in one semester. Others, away from the day-to-day assistance of parents and family for the first time in their lives, become overwhelmed with the number of decisions and choices facing them.

Tips for College Success

To ensure your college experience is a positive one, make sure you plan ahead. Address your inherent limitations and map out a plan of action to deal with them. Make sure you have access to learning services and academic support to help reduce stress and frustration.

If you have significant problems with executive functions, hire an ADHD coach who can help you organize your time and establish good study habits. Joining an ADHD support group or peer study group on campus may lead to meaningful friendships, help you feel more hooked into campus life, and give you a safe place to vent your fears and frustrations. If the college has a student health center, introduce yourself to the physician on staff.

If you're taking ADHD medications, ask your physician about extending them throughout the day by giving you multiple doses of the same medication or long- and short-acting medications. You'll also want to make sure your medication isn't prescribed in a way that would interfere with your sleep.

When ADHD Is "All in the Family"

Given the genetic component of ADHD, there's a 50 percent chance that, if you or your spouse has adult ADHD, one or more of your children will have it. According to research by the NIH, mental health problems in parents can interfere with a child's treatment and recovery because treatments for children with ADHD rely heavily on parental support. In addition, parents of children with ADHD are three times more likely to separate or divorce as parents of children without the disorder.

Here are a few pointers that may help keep things sane when multiple family members have ADHD:

❏ Make sure the entire family is as informed as possible about ADHD. Attend meetings, seminars, and workshops together, and join support groups for families with ADHD for first-hand advice on how to handle specific situations.

❏ Be realistic. Instead of trying to conform to what you think is "normal" family life, embrace the many gifts that come with ADHD and find ways for individual family members to shine.

❏ Make sure everyone in the family who wants or needs professional help gets counseling, therapy, or coaching. Consider individual, family, and couples counseling to keep things running smoothly. Studies show that families cope best with ADHD when they use several different types of therapy.

❏ Be thoroughly acquainted with the many types of disability benefits, specialized instruction, technology, and financial resources at your disposal. This is especially important if you have children with ADHD heading to college.

❏ Laughter can be the best medicine. Don't be afraid to find the humor in snafus that arise at home. Finding the lighter side of things can help both parents and children have more patience, forgiveness, and flexibility when dealing with ADHD.

Adult ADHD in the Elderly

Although there is very little research on adult ADHD in the elderly, a high percentage of adults with the disorder will still have the condition as they head into their golden years. By the time they reach their senior years, adults with ADHD may also suffer from other medical problems or diseases—including dementia, Alzheimer's disease, diabetes, heart conditions, and cancer—which may mimic or mask the symptoms of ADHD.

Prescription Drugs and the Elderly

Although people over age 65 make up just 13 percent of the U.S. population, they account for 30 percent of prescription drug prescriptions. Many seniors are very sensitive to drugs, may eliminate them more slowly, and may require lower or less frequent dosages. Because of forgetfulness and memory problems, they may also take too much medication accidentally. The use of weekly or monthly pill boxes can be a great memory aid for seniors suffering from adult ADHD.

Fact

Early research indicates that Ritalin, a drug prescribed for adult ADHD, may help prevent falls in the elderly and in patients with Parkinson's disease. Although the study was too small to warrant the widespread prescription of Ritalin, its results suggest that treating cognitive defects associated with aging and diseases like ADHD may decrease falls in the elderly.

If you suspect that you or a senior citizen you love is suffering from adult ADHD, a medical expert who specializes in gerontology can help distinguish common diseases and/or normal signs of aging from the symptoms of adult ADHD.

CHAPTER 5

Understanding Diagnostic Challenges and Limitations

A dult ADHD is nearly always difficult to diagnose. Research shows that between 50 and 70 percent of people with ADHD suffer from overlapping, associated, or comorbid conditions such as clinical anxiety, depression, learning disorders, bipolar disorder, and substance abuse.

The Problem with Comorbid Conditions

Adults with ADHD have a high incidence of coexisting or comorbid conditions, according to the 2004 National Comorbidity Survey, which studied the entire U.S. population between the ages of fifteen and forty-five. This research showed that 45 percent of adults with ADHD had mood disorders, including depression. Those rates were three times the instance of depression in the general population. In addition, 59 percent suffered from anxiety disorders (3.2 times higher than the general population), 35 percent had issues with substance or alcohol abuse or dependency (2.8 times the general population), and 69 percent suffered from impulse disorders (5.9 times the general population). Other research showed that adults with varying types of ADHD had an even higher rate of coexisting conditions than did children with ADHD.

Among adults with the combined type of ADHD, 69 percent had some history of substance abuse and dependence. In addition, at some point in their lives 63 percent had been treated for depression, 35 percent for anxiety, and 30 percent for conduct disorders. Studies show that more than a third of adults with ADHD also suffer from oppositional disorder at some time in their life, and nearly a quarter of them suffer from social phobia.

Executive Function Impairments

Adults with ADHD are also highly likely to suffer from a wide variety of executive function impairments that can impact every area of their lives. Put another way, the brain of an adult with ADHD can be compared to a computer with an erratic operating system that interferes with running the essential software they need to succeed at work, at home, and in their relationships.

Cluster Theory of Adult ADHD

Why 88 percent of adults with ADIID—six times the rate of the general population—suffer from some type of psychiatric condition is a factor that continues to puzzle scientists. Some experts attribute it to genetics and the fact that people simply inherit a particular form of psychiatric problems. Others believe the answer may stem from a theory holding that ADHD is not one disorder, but a complicated syndrome made up of a cluster of impairments that affects many different parts of the brain, and which causes or contributes to many different types of psychiatric illnesses.

Confusing Symptoms of Stress and Depression for Adult ADHD

If you suffer from depression and stress, you're not alone: more than 17 million Americans of all ages, races, and socioeconomic backgrounds experience depression.

If you're an adult with ADHD, research shows that you have three times the risk of suffering from major depression, and more than seven times the risk of suffering from dysthymia, or chronic low-level depression.

Researchers believe depression is more common among adults with ADHD because the same neurobiological systems in the brain that control mood also control attention. Another prominent theory holds that the relationship between ADHD and depression may result from the many social and interpersonal difficulties experienced by children and adults with the disorder.

Is It Depression or Adult ADHD?

It takes a professional familiar with both conditions to differentiate between depression and adult ADHD. Both are marked by moodiness, forgetfulness, an inability to pay attention, a lack of motivation, and feelings of helplessness and hopelessness. Complicating matters is the fact that many medications used to treat adult ADHD may also increase symptoms of depression. Although it can be hard to generalize, experts say, people suffering from depression tend to feel dark and gloomy for weeks or months at a time, while people suffering from adult ADHD are more likely to experience transient feelings of depression in response to specific situation or setbacks.

Fact

While no one is sure why adults with ADHD tend to be moody, grumpy, depressed, and pessimistic, scientists today believe the ADHD "downer personality" may be the result of neurological dysfunctions in the brain combined with a patient's emotional response to repeated failure, frustration, and disappointment in life.

Another marked difference between depression and adult ADHD is that people who are clinically depressed usually don't have the energy to make a move. Adults with ADHD, on the other hand, often feel too overwhelmed or befuddled to know what to do first.

There are also some subtle differences in the way depression and adult ADHD affect sleep. While both conditions cause insomnia, depressed people usually fall asleep easily but awaken several times a night with anxious, racing thoughts. Adults with ADHD, on the other hand, often have trouble falling asleep because their minds are racing or they are obsessing about something.

Primary and Secondary Depression

Primary depression appears to strike out of nowhere and lingers for weeks or months. Unlike secondary depression, it also appears to be an inherited disorder. Secondary depression is usually a response to the sort of chronic failures, disappointments, and frustrations many adults with ADHD routinely experience at work, in their marriage and friendships, and in social situations.

Depression and Seasonal Affective Disorder

Seasonal affective disorder (SAD) is a mood disorder associated with depression and related to seasonal variations in light. SAD affects up to 20 percent of the population living in states with harsh winter conditions, and may disproportionately affect adults with ADHD. SAD is believed to be caused by an overproduction of melatonin, a sleep-related hormone secreted by the brain at increased levels in the dark and believed to cause symptoms of depression. The most difficult months for adults with ADHD are January and February, and younger people and women appear to be at higher risk. Treatment to suppress the brain's secretion of melatonin ranges from phototherapy, or bright light therapy, to spending more time outdoors during daylight hours.

The Many Faces of Adult Depression

Like adult ADHD, adult depression is not a one-size-fits-all illness. Clinical depression is the broad-based definition for any depression severe enough to warrant treatment. Clinical depression is also called unipolar depression, major depression, severe depression, or major depressive disorder. Dysthymia is chronic, low-level depression that just won't lift.

Atypical depression often affects women and is characterized by periods of depression that appear to improve but then get worse. Types of atypical depression include overeating, eating disorders, panic attacks, hypersensitivity, and oversleeping.

Bipolar disorder, or manic depression, is marked by roller-coaster highs and lows. The condition is caused by an imbalance in brain chemicals.

How Depression Affects Women

Major and minor depression affects twice as many women as men, regardless of whether or not they also have adult ADHD. Although women are more likely to seek medical help, they are also more prone to blame themselves for the condition and withdraw from society. Here are some key reasons why depression rates are higher in women than men.

- Women are twice as likely to be depressed because of social factors such as physical and sexual abuse, domestic violence, poverty, and single parenthood.
- Research by the NIMH indicates that women are more vulnerable to "life stresses" that contribute to depression, including sexual discrimination at work, increased workloads, and family responsibilities.
- About 10 percent of new mothers suffer from postpartum depression, a type of depression caused by wildly fluctuating hormones after pregnancy. Half of all new mothers experience this milder form of depression.
- Many women suffer from PMS, which includes mild depression and bloating. Premenstrual dysphoric disorder (PMDD), a more serious condition, affects about 4 percent of women and results in severe irritability and depression for up to two

weeks prior to or during menstruation. Studies show that, because of underlying hormonal changes, women with PMDD are more likely to suffer from depression later in life.

- Infertility and miscarriage may contribute to depression in women.
- Taking oral contraceptives has been linked to depression in women.

Menopause is another leading cause of depression in women; the dramatic drop in estrogen before, during, and after menopause is to blame. As levels of estrogen decrease, women may have trouble sleeping, experience sexual problems, have annoying hot flashes, have problems maintaining an ideal weight, and suffer from low self-esteem and body image. Lower levels of estrogen can also weaken bones and cause thinning of the hair and skin.

As if that's not enough, for many women menopause coincides with retirement, divorce, or empty nest syndrome and could trigger feelings of mortality. Societal emphasis on youth and beauty can also make it difficult for women going through menopause to feel attractive, worthwhile, or desirable.

Men and Depression

More than 6 million American men are treated for depression every year, but the condition is still undertreated. Blame it on societal standards, but men typically deny or mask their feelings with alcohol, drugs, or by overworking. Because a man's sense of worth is closely tied to his work, many men experience depression after being laid off or fired, especially if they don't have concrete career goals or aspirations.

Male menopause, or midlife crisis, usually affects men between the ages of thirty-five and fifty. A man suffering from a midlife crisis and depression is often discontented and bored with a life that once felt happy and fulfilling.

Depression in Young Adults

Moodiness and adolescence often go hand-in-hand, making the diagnosis of depression and adult ADHD particularly difficult. Studies indicate that as many as one in five teenagers may be depressed. Unfortunately, depression in teenagers is a serious condition and suicide is the third-leading cause of death for adolescents ages fifteen to nineteen.

Symptoms of teenage depression include agitation, restlessness, anger, rage, indecision, hopelessness, helplessness, feelings of guilt, and an inability to concentrate. Failing grades, withdrawing from friends and family, changes in sleep habits, eating disorders, and suicidal thoughts or actions are other tell-tale signs.

Depression in Senior Citizens

About 6 million Americans are aged sixty-five and older, and one in three of them suffer from depression. Geriatric depression is particularly common among people who are widowed, living alone, have alcohol or substance abuse problems, live with chronic pain, or have a prior history of depression. Seniors taking a combination of drugs may experience depression as a side effect.

Other factors that may trigger geriatric depression include being diagnosed with a serious illness or a loss of independence, such as losing a driver's license or moving to a nursing home. Symptoms of geriatric depression include insomnia, decreased appetite, social withdrawal, and thoughts of suicide or attempted suicide. Geriatric depression may also lower a person's immunity and make her more susceptible to infection and disease. Unfortunately, 90 percent of seniors suffering from depression are never diagnosed or treated. Some suffer from dementia or other types of mental conditions that have similar symptoms to depressions. Others don't tell family members they are depressed because they fear it could ultimately lead to placement in a managed care facility.

Treat Depression, Adult ADHD, or Both?

For years, medical science believed depression was a natural by-product of living with the disappointments and setbacks of adult ADHD. If adult ADHD were treated, depression would also be alleviated. With that theory in mind, physicians considered adult ADHD the primary diagnosis and took no additional steps to treat the depression.

But recent studies at Massachusetts General Hospital in Boston established depression and adult ADHD as separate conditions that require separate treatments. Today, some medical experts prefer to get depression under control before treating adult ADHD. In this case, depression becomes the primary disorder and adult ADHD is the secondary condition. Other experts prefer to treat both conditions simultaneously in the belief that both disorders must be managed before either one is under control.

Research shows that medications for depression work equally well for adults with and without ADHD.

Challenges in Diagnosing Women with ADHD

Until recently, adult ADHD was a silent disorder in women that was routinely ignored or misdiagnosed by the educational and medical community. To address the millions of girls and women suffering in silence, the National Center for Girls and Women with AD/HD was founded in 1997 to promote awareness and research on ADHD in women. Unfortunately, according to the organization, current diagnostic criteria continue to emphasize traits common to boys and leave the majority of girls and women out of the equation. Even when a woman believes she has adult ADHD, very few clinicians are equipped or have the experience or background to diagnose and treat her. Because there are no specific criteria for treating women, most medical experts continue to rely on standard psychotherapeutic approaches that may provide women with helpful insights into their emotional and personal issues, but often fail to give them the tools and strategies they need to manage the condition on a daily basis and lead a more productive life.

Because so few studies have been conducted on women and ADHD, and women have only recently begun to be diagnosed and treated, most of what we know is based on the clinical experience of mental health professionals who have specialized in treating women. While research on women with adult ADHD still lags behind that of adult males, medical experts are beginning to discover some major differences in their coexisting conditions and symptoms.

Coexisting Conditions and Symptoms of Women

Depression, anxiety, low self-image, compulsive eating, eating disorders, alcohol abuse, and chronic sleep deprivation are just a few of many comorbid conditions that may be present in women with ADHD. While women with ADHD experience the same rates of depression and anxiety disorders as men with ADHD, studies show women also tend to have a higher degree of psychological distress and a lower self-image than men with ADHD.

Alert

Unlike men, women with adult ADHD tend to attribute their successes and failure to outside factors like fate, luck, and chance rather than to personal factors like effort, drive, and talent. Women are also more likely to use coping measures to reduce or manage ADHD-related stress than to take direct action to alleviate it.

Women diagnosed with ADHD in adulthood also have more depressive symptoms and are more stressed out and anxious than women without the disorder. New studies also show that stress levels may be higher for women suffering from adult ADHD than men, because women tend to feel more responsibility for the home, children, and family. They also suffer more chronic stress, and are at an increased risk for diseases related to stress, including migraines, cancer, and fibromyalgia.

Medication Management and Women

Prescribing the right medication in the right dosage is another challenge facing experts who treat women with ADHD. Because adult ADHD symptoms tend to flare when estrogen levels decline, the natural fluctuation of hormones within the menstrual cycle, in pregnant and postpartum women, and in menopausal women can exacerbate symptoms.

Poverty and Adult ADHD

Researchers are just beginning to study and predict the impact of childhood variables on the risk of developing adult ADHD. According to one study, the four most powerful positive variables predicting a good outcome for children include being raised in an intact household above the poverty level, by parents who don't have psychiatric problems, with a consistent parenting style, and by parents who are emotionally and physically available to their children.

Studies also show that aggressive behavior, depression, and substance abuse on the part of parents may increase their children's risk of adult ADHD. Other variables likely to increase the risks include parental psychopathy, learning disabilities, and lower intellect.

Research also shows that children and teenagers raised in poverty have a higher chance of having parents who are either unemployed or underemployed, lack health insurance, and do not schedule regular medical checkups for either their children or themselves. If one or both parents has adult ADHD, the chances are even higher that a child will be brought up in poverty because his parent(s) may be unable to get or keep jobs, are at a higher risk of getting divorced, and are also more likely to be arrested and jailed.

CHAPTER 6

Meet the Screening Tests

G etting a diagnosis for adult ADHD can be challenging for everyone involved. Because there is no lab test that provides diagnostic certainty, physicians must use a variety of tools and piece together a diagnosis like a puzzle. They rely on professional observations and information gleaned from a physical exam, patient interviews, school reports, test results and job evaluations, and blood tests to rule out conditions with similar symptoms, such as thyroid disease. Other tests and evaluations can determine if learning disorders or neurological problems are involved.

Types of Medical Specialists
Who Treat Adult ADHD

Many people don't know where to begin when they suspect they may have adult ADHD. Unlike diseases and conditions that can be easily diagnosed with a blood test or an X-ray, there is no one simple test that confirms ADHD. For most adults, getting the right diagnosis usually entails a series of assessments from one or more medical professionals. In fact, many experts believe the best diagnostic and treatment plan is a multidisciplinary approach that involves a team of various medical and adult ADHD experts. Before beginning your search for a medical professional who can diagnose and treat you, it helps to understand the different strengths and limitations of the various types of medical care.

Your Family Doctor

Many adults with ADHD feel most comfortable beginning with their family physician, if only because she may be more familiar with them from a personal and medical perspective than anyone else. But as with any medical specialist, there are several pros and cons to weigh.

Since you can't be diagnosed with adult ADHD until it's already been established that you had it as a child, it may be easier for your family physician, if she has known you since you were a child, to arrive at a diagnosis than a physician who has never met you before.

Your family physician can also order the necessary medical tests and procedures you may require, and she can also prescribe prescription drugs. It may also be easier to see your family physician than it would be to see a specialist who doesn't know you, and she is likely to charge less than some specialists.

On the other hand, your family physician may not have the expertise or experience in diagnosing and treating adult ADHD as a specialist would, although family physicians are becoming increasingly aware of the condition. In addition, she may not be comfortable diagnosing a condition in which a common treatment is the long-term use of stimulant drugs. Also, she may not be able to adequately address a complicated disorder like adult ADHD in the time span of a normal office visit.

Psychiatrists or Psychologists?

While both psychiatrists and psychologists deal with mental and emotional disorders, they are likely to approach diagnosis and treatment in different ways. As medical doctors, psychiatrists can prescribe medical tests and medications. But they may or may not be trained or interested in counseling or be able to assist you in dealing with practical, everyday problems associated with adult ADHD. Psychiatrists tend to be more expensive than psychologists, charging

$200 and up for a 45-minute to hour-long session. Depending on their discipline, some psychiatrists, such as psychoanalysts, often require that patients make a long-term commitment to therapy.

Psychologists are not medical doctors, but they are highly trained in the workings of the mind, as well as in the areas of counseling and diagnosis.

Many adults with ADHD find psychologists invaluable in helping them find new and better ways to cope with everyday issues and problems related to the disorder. They may also view their psychologist as a confidant with whom they can safely discuss personal or professional issues. A psychologist must refer patients to medical doctors for prescriptions and some medical tests. Most psychologists charge less than psychiatrists.

Fact

Your psychologist may use a variety of nonmedical tests to arrive at a diagnosis. These may include tests for learning disabilities and adult intelligence, tests for educational achievement, IQ tests, and tests for memory, information processing, and auditory discrimination. Many psychologists also use computerized tests like IVA-Plus to measure a multitude of auditory and visual performance skills.

Neuropsychologists are trained in the biological and neurological basis of thought and learning. They may use a battery of tests to measure cognitive and behavioral functioning.

A neuropsychologist can use these tests as the basis for making recommendations about your overall treatment, and diagnosing learning abilities that may be hindering your performance at work or school. Tests may also be administered to establish a legal basis for disability services, or to protect your rights at work or in college. Neuropsychologists are usually less expensive than psychiatrists, but more expensive than psychologists.

Neurologists

Neurologists are medical doctors who specialize in diagnosing and treating diseases and disorders of the brain and nervous system. Neurologists may be able to differentiate between symptoms of adult ADHD and overlapping conditions like seizure disorder or brain injury. They can also prescribe medications and medical tests. Unfortunately, they tend to be very expensive.

Psychiatric Nurse Practitioners and Nurse Practitioners

Psychiatric nurse practitioners are generally well trained and knowledgeable about the diagnosis and treatment of adult ADHD.

Registered nurses, or RNs, may also be able to make an initial diagnosis and offer assistance with life skills. As with psychiatric nurses, they can't prescribe medical tests or medications and must refer patients to medical professionals. They are, however, usually less expensive and easier to schedule than psychologists or psychiatrists.

Other Types of Specialists

In addition to psychiatrists and psychologists, there are many other types of specialists who diagnose and help treat adult ADHD and who may be able to offer additional assistance with assessment, coping skills, behavioral modification, and problem solving.

Master and Doctoral Level Counselors

Provided they have the appropriate training, they can do an initial assessment and help you deal with a wide variety of everyday life skills and problems. However, they must refer you to a doctor or another professional for medication and medical testing. They may also provide services like neurofeedback and biofeedback. Individual, group, family, and marriage counselors and therapists can provide help in dealing with specific issues like getting along in social settings, functioning at work, parenting, organizational issues at home, and dealing with adult ADHD-related problems in relationships and marriage.

Social Workers

Social workers are usually employed by public or private health care agencies to offer counseling. Treatment is generally affordable. While social workers may be able to offer an initial diagnosis, they often lack the training necessary to distinguish between the symptoms of adult ADHD and overlapping conditions like clinical depression, anxiety, or bipolar disorder.

Adult ADHD Coaches

One of the fastest-growing resources for adults with ADHD is in the area of ADHD coaching. Coaches specialize in helping people manage everyday problems and situations, such as organization, time management, memory, follow-through, and motivation. Unlike psychiatrists and psychologists, they don't give advice or counsel, nor are they concerned with delving into or rehashing past mistakes, setbacks, or negative experiences. Instead, they address the present, using an approach that asks clients to focus on where they are now, where they want to be, and how they can get there.

Alert

Unlike doctors, coaches are not licensed by regulatory boards, nor are they required to undergo special training or licensing to practice. For this reason, some medical professionals question the validity of coaching as supplemental therapy. For more information on accredited coaches in your area, visit the International Coaching Federation website at *www.coachfederation.org*.

Support Groups and Online Resources

If you have adult ADHD, it may be a good idea to join an adult ADHD support group in your community. Ask your therapist if she has suggestions on local support groups to join, or go to CHADD's website (*www.chadd.org*) for a list of support groups throughout the country. You can also call your local college or university mental health counselor for suggestions.

Support groups can provide you with information on recommended physicians, specialists, and treatments in your areas, and may also offer you the moral support you need. Online resources can be a convenient way to access up-to-date information and resources on adult ADHD.

Overview of Initial Evaluations Your Doctor May Use

If an adult was not diagnosed with ADHD as a child, the doctor must establish a childhood diagnosis.

If a physician can't make a definitive diagnosis based on a developmental history, or if the described symptoms don't exactly match the profile of adult ADHD, he may order additional tests to fill in the blanks. Experts dispute the effectiveness of these tests, but the test manufacturers claim their tests can do everything from pinpoint the causes of emotional and behavioral problems to predict what treatment will work best.

 Alert

To date, there are no neuropsychological tests that reliably identify adult ADHD. Although cognitive tests may point to deficiencies in some people with the disorder, this is not true in all cases. Complicating the picture is the fact that some adults who have low scores for impulsivity do not meet criteria for adult ADHD.

While some experts place a lot of faith in tests, the general consensus among physicians who treat adult ADHD is that, while tests can be useful tools, there is not enough evidence to indicate that tests can be used to accurately diagnose specific cases of adult ADHD.

Rating Scales

Rating scales give physicians a structure in which to gather symptom-related information and provide a large volume of valuable data in a short amount of time to facilitate diagnosis.

While many medical experts consider rating scales to be the most accurate method of diagnosing adult ADHD, they are not 100 percent accurate. Rating scales rely heavily on a patient's ability to remember childhood symptoms and can't conclusively prove that symptoms have persisted since childhood, a major criterion of adult ADHD. They are most useful when used in combination with physician-patient interviews, developmental histories, and other corroborating evidence. There are three types of rating scales: screening tests that identify adults at risk for adult ADHD, symptom assessment scales that can be self-administered or given by your doctor, and formal diagnostic scales.

Screening Tests

The most popular screening test is the adult ADHD self-report scale, which queries patients about eighteen symptoms of adult ADHD and has them rate these symptoms on a five-point scale that ranges from "Never" to "Often."

Patients are asked questions relating to problems completing tasks, remembering appointments, fidgeting and squirming, procrastinating, making careless mistakes, having trouble paying attention, misplacing things, being distracted, talking too much in social situations, interrupting people or butting in, and having problems relaxing and unwinding.

Symptom Assessment Scales

Symptom assessment scales were developed to assess current adult ADHD symptoms. Some are clinician-administered, while others can be administered by the doctor or patient. While some deal with the eighteen core symptoms of adult ADHD, others look at additional symptoms, including problems with executive functions and mood swings.

Some tests use "prompts" or questions to get patients to discuss their disorder. Questions relate to making mistakes at school or work, having trouble with details, having difficulty staying focused while reading, watching movies or attending lectures, and feeling wired and unable to slow down and relax. Commonly used scales include the Brown ADD Scale, the Conners Adult ADHD Rating Scale, the Wender-Reimherr ADHD Scale, the ADHD Rating Scale, and the Adult Investigator Symptom Report Scale.

Diagnostic Scales

Clinicians use diagnostic scales to establish and document the presence and severity of childhood symptoms of ADHD and the severity and impact of adult ADHD symptoms. The most commonly used adult ADHD diagnostic scales are the Conners' Adult ADHD Diagnostic Interview, the Barkley Current Symptoms Scale, the Brown ADD Scale, the Kiddie-SADS Diagnostic Interview ADHD module, and the Adult ADHD Clinician Diagnostic Scale.

Continuous Performance Tests

A relative newcomer to the ADHD testing mix, continuous performance tests (CPT) are computerized tests used to measure attention and impulse control. During the test, which lasts about twenty minutes, the patient performs a simple task, like pressing a button as quickly as possible, whenever she sees a certain letter or image appear on the screen (for instance, an "X" that appears in a rapid succession of images).

To increase the difficulty, some tests change the task so that the person must only click if they see the letter "A" before the letter "X." Other tests may use numbers, symbols, or even sounds, but the basic task uses the same concept.

Alert

Medical experts remain divided about the diagnostic usefulness of CPTs. Some physicians feel that CPTs provide too many false positives and negatives to be useful at all. Others believe the information provided by the tests is useful, but only if viewed in a larger context of other relevant data.

CPTs can be administered by psychologists, social workers, physicians, counselors, psychiatric workers, pediatric nurses, teachers, and school officials. They are typically given in schools, outpatient and inpatient clinics, residential treatment centers, child protective services, special education and regular classrooms, juvenile detention centers, and private practice offices.

The Test of Variables of Attention (TOVA)

One of the most widely used CPTs is the TOVA, an objective, neurophysiological measure of attention rather than a subjective rating behavior. The twenty-one-minute test is a very simple, standardized, computer gamelike exam that measures responses to either visual or auditory stimuli. These measurements are then compared to the measurements of a group of people without attention disorders who took the TOVA.

The TOVA tests for both visual and auditory attention because most people are "concordant" for both visual and auditory information processing, meaning they process visual and aural information similarly. Twelve percent of people are "discordant" and process visual or auditory information differently, or are significantly slower in one modality than the other. Unlike some CPTs, the TOVA avoids the confusing effects of language, cultural differences, learning problems, memory, and processing complex sequences.

Fact

Proponents of the TOVA claim the test is long enough, simple enough, and boring enough to be relatively accurate. It's long enough to catch those individuals with ADHD who can rise to the occasion and do all the right things with shorter CPTs. Instead of using the complex, sequential targets that other CPTs do, it keeps the same boring presentation interval.

Because the TOVA comes in a clinical and screening version, it can be used in a wide variety of clinical and nonclinical settings. The clinical version is used by licensed clinicians, while the screening version of the test can be used in nonclinical settings such as schools, human resource departments, and rehabilitation programs. Any personnel can be trained to administer the screening version. The only difference between the two tests is that the screening version has no diagnostic terms in the report and summarizes results as either within normal range or not within normal range. Results of the TOVA are immediately available.

The Conners' Continuous Performance Test

Another popular computerized CPT is the Conners' Continuous Performance Test. Test response patterns provide information that enables the practitioner to better understand the type of deficits that might be present. For example, some response patterns suggest inattentiveness or impulsivity, while other response patterns may indicate activation/arousal problems or difficulties maintaining vigilance.

Neuropsychological Testing

Neuropsychology is the study of how the functions of your brain and nervous system affect the way you think and behave. For years, neuropsychology has been used by hospital clinicians to assess patients with head injuries to determine how neurological damage might affect their thinking skills or behavior.

Clinical psychologists have also used it to more accurately assess the causes of some patients' behavior. More recently, education experts have begun using neuropsychology to explain why some children have trouble acquiring language, mathematical reasoning, and reading skills.

How Neuropsychological Testing Works

Neuropsychological testing measures a patient's cognitive abilities, memory, and motor skills. It may be helpful in distinguishing between adult ADHD and comorbid conditions, and between adult ADHD and learning disabilities. Neuropsychological tests can also examine attention (verbal and written as well as sustained and variable), impulse control, recall, memory, reaction time, processing speed, executive functions, working memory, and a person's awareness of his environment. They may also include intelligence and achievement assessments.

Pros and Cons

Neuropsychological testing can provide useful data. But research shows that neuropsychological tests fail to pick up deficits in one third to one half of all adults who take them.

Intellectual and Memory Tests

Adults with ADHD tend to be weaker in areas requiring more focused attention, such as making mathematical computations and recognizing patterns. The Wechsler Adult Intelligence Scale

(WAIS) is widely used in the diagnosis of adult ADHD. The test measures two broad areas of intelligence, including verbal skills and performance skills.

It also assesses factual knowledge, spatial skills, logical thinking, and mathematical ability. The results of both tests are combined for the IQ score, which can be used to compare adults with ADHD to adults without the disorder.

Memory Tests

Memory is a process rather than a specific part of the brain. It functions as a system with many parts scattered throughout the brain. While adults with ADHD don't necessarily have bad memories, they do have unique symptoms that may create gaps in their memory processes. For instance, since adults with the disorder usually need to be motivated and interested to acquire knowledge, they may only remember information they deem fascinating and dump valuable details that may be boring.

The Wechsler Memory Scale is often used to test memory strengths and weaknesses in adults with ADHD. The scale is a battery of memory tests that consists of eleven subtests, including six primary and five optional subtests. The primary subtests test logical memory (like remembering a story), verbal paired associates (remembering word sets), letter-number sequencing, and tasks related to visual memory. Optional subtests test information and orientation, and memory for lists of words and numbers.

Blood and Laboratory Tests for Adult ADHD

Although there are no blood or laboratory tests that diagnose adult ADHD, physicians may use various tests to rule out conditions that have symptoms in common with adult ADHD. One simple and inexpensive blood test your doctor is likely to order will check your thyroid hormone levels. Abnormal thyroid levels are very common in women over age fifty and are often mistaken for adult ADHD.

Your doctor may also order tests that measure your Serum CBC count with differential and your electrolyte levels. In general, adult ADHD patients undergo liver function tests before starting stimulant drugs for adult ADHD, the most common type of medication prescribed for the disorder, to ensure their livers are healthy enough to handle the medications.

Brain Scans and Imaging

The evidence seems to favor using brain imaging to help diagnose and treat adult ADHD, but medical experts remain divided about its current overall effectiveness. Although brain imaging tests can't provide a definite diagnosis, they do offer a wealth of data that can be compared to databases on thousands of other patients with adult ADHD.

MRI

Brain imaging, or MRI, produces a clear, detailed picture of brain structures. An MRI can show slight variations between the brains of people with ADHD and those without it.

A functional MRI, or an FMRI, is a more powerful type of MRI that analyzes brain activity. Unfortunately, it's so new that many radiologists haven't been trained to use it yet.

PET Scans

Positron emission topography (PET) scans measure the presence and motion of radioactive substances that are injected into a patient. As the radioactive material travels to the brain, the PET shows blood flow and glucose metabolism. As part of a growing field of high-tech medicine called nuclear medicine, PET scans provide very high-quality images of the brain that far surpass what older devices can do.

SPECT scans

SPECT scans are a lower-tech version of PET scans. It's still the same basic scenario: radioactive substances are injected into the arm and provide a record of what happens as the material travels to the brain. These scans are less detailed than those recorded by PET scans, but SPECT scans cost much less than PET scans, are easier to administer, and are more widely available.

EEG

Electroencephalogram technology, or EEG, measures the electrical activity in your brain, otherwise known as brain waves. Electrodes placed on the scalp transmit information about brain waves to an amplifying device, then on to a computer so a neurologist can view and analyze them. It's been useful in showing an increase in larger, slower brain waves, which some researchers believe is an indication of ADHD. The downside to EEG is that it only tracks brain waves on the surface of the brain and can't see into the organ like newer technology.

QEEG

Quantitative Electroencephalogram, or QEEG, measures brain wave activity against normal brain waves stored in a database.

ERP

Event-related potential (ERP) tests record changes in brain activity via electrodes placed on the scalp. Changes are measured against a repeated stimulus. People with ADHD often respond to the stimulus in a certain way that confirms or aids diagnosis.

CHAPTER 7

How You Can Help
Your Doctor

Although ADHD sometimes isn't discovered until adulthood, the disorder always begins in childhood and never spontaneously develops in adults. According to current diagnostic criteria, adults can't be diagnosed with adult ADHD unless it can be established they have had the disorder since they were at least seven years old. If you suspect you have adult ADHD but were never diagnosed as a child, it's possible for your medical experts to make a retrospective diagnosis through clinical interviews, physical examinations, and tests.

Developing a History of Behavior

Your physician will probably begin his analysis with a diagnostic review during which he will gather information about your developmental history, health history, school history, employment history, social history, childhood and present behavior patterns, alcohol and drug history, and psychiatric history. He will also conduct a complete medical interview to rule out other medical conditions to which ADHD may be secondary or whose symptoms may mask or mimic adult ADHD.

Since adult ADHD often includes neuropsychological problems, he may also administer or prescribe tests that measure attention, memory, intellectual functioning, and academic achievement. Test scores, as well as your response to taking tests, can help determine if your symptoms demonstrate ADHD.

Patient Interviews

Your physician will also conduct clinical interviews with you, your parents, teachers, and friends who knew you as a child to find out more about your behavior then. As you might imagine, trying to remember specific details of your behavior more than twenty, thirty, or even forty years ago can be daunting. In addition, studies have cast doubt on the validity of using personal memories to establish a backward diagnosis of adult ADHD, claiming many childhood memories are too inaccurate or subjective to be clinically relevant.

In fact, a growing number of adult ADHD experts are pushing for the creation and adoption of new adult criteria that would advance the onset of ADHD from age seven to between the ages of sixteen to eighteen. New criteria would also place much less importance on childhood memories in establishing a diagnosis. But until ADHD diagnostic criteria are reviewed and possibly revised in 2012, patients and experts alike are hampered by the current guidelines.

Parents and Teacher Interviews

Although teachers are often the first to suggest that a child has ADHD, parents are usually the first to suspect a child has a problem.

Essential

A medical expert needs to be a great detective to assemble a valuable history of behavior. She must know enough about childhood and adult ADHD to ask relevant questions, gather and interpret a wide range of data, and weigh recollections against objective facts.

Unfortunately, studies show that recollections from parents and teachers regarding the childhood behavior of an adult are usually much less accurate than memories provided by patients.

Genetic Factors

Because ADHD has a strong genetic component, a history of ADHD in the immediate or extended family may be useful in determining the childhood status of an adult patient.

Fact

As an adopted child, Ruth always suspected something was wrong, but she had no family medical history to reference. After tracking down and meeting her biological family, the forty-seven-year-old learned that her biological parents and her three biological siblings had ADHD. In fact, all three siblings had suffered experiences similar to hers in college, and had "fallen apart and dropped out."

Parents of children with ADHD are twenty-four times as likely to suffer from the disorder themselves as are parents of children without the disorder, according to a study in the *Journal of the American Academy of Child & Adolescent Psychiatry.* Parents whose children had both ADHD and oppositional defiant disorder or conduct disorder were found more likely to have mood, anxiety, and substance abuse issues than other parents. Living with kids who have ADHD can also exacerbate a parent's own problems, and vice versa.

Family and Personal Medical History

Understanding your personal health and your family's health history is another important part of the diagnosis, especially if your symptoms came on recently—a strong indication you are suffering from a condition other than adult ADHD. Your doctor may administer or prescribe a psychiatric and medical exam to look for diseases and conditions that may impact your ability to pay attention and focus, or which may cause you to feel and act hyperactive and impulsive. These may include learning disabilities, hyperthyroidism, hypothyroidism, fetal alcohol syndrome, depression, and anxiety.

Other Childhood Illness That May Have an Impact on ADHD

Your medical expert will also probably review your childhood medical records for evidence of diseases and conditions that are often linked with ADHD.

- Vision and hearing problems may also cause or masquerade as ADHD in childhood. Recent studies show that children with convergence insufficiency, a physical eye problem that makes it hard to keep both eyes pointed and focused at a near target, are three times as likely to be diagnosed with ADHD than children without the disorder.
- Central Auditory Processing Disorder (CAPD) will sometimes occur in children who have had a history of ear infections and/or PE tubes. Symptoms include distractibility, inability to follow a set of verbal instructions, and spacing out.
- Yeast infections cause hyperactivity in children. Most children who suffer from yeast infections have some underlying problem that is frequently traced to an immune disorder or a disorder affecting carbohydrate metabolism that alters blood sugar levels. In yeast infections, intestinal parasites rob the body of needed nutrients, which in turn affects behavior.
- Streptococcus bacteria, better known as strep, can cause rheumatic fever and a movement disorder known as Sydenham's chorea if left untreated. Recurrent infections can also lead to a group of symptoms collectively known as PANDAS (pediatric autoimmune neuropsychiatric disorders). Some symptoms of PANDAS include obsessive-compulsive behav-

ior, Tourette's syndrome, hyperactivity, cognitive problems, and fidgeting.

- Hypoglycemia, or low blood sugar, can stem from thyroid disorders, liver or pancreatic problems, adrenal gland abnormalities, or insufficient diet.
- Head injuries such as post-concussion syndrome have symptoms that include irritability, mood swings, memory problems, depression, and sleeping problems.
- Some spinal problems can cause ADHD-like behavior. If the spine is not connected to the brain properly, nerves from the spinal cord can give the brain all of the signals at once and cause a child to be hyperactive.
- Some drugs can cause the brain to atrophy, leading to disturbed cognition and behavior. If a child routinely takes prescription or over-the-counter medications for asthma, hay fever, allergies, headaches, or any other condition, medication may cause or contribute to behavior problems.
- Sniffing materials such as modeling glue or other household products can cause hyperactivity and inattention.

Your physician will gather information on your personal and family medical history, including records of allergies, asthma, tics, epilepsy, or other medical conditions, and a history of your major developmental milestones, such as when you first crawled, walked, spoke, and read. He will also inquire about psychiatric disease, depression, alcoholism, and substance abuse in your family history.

Coexisting Conditions That Mimic ADHD

Most children and adults with ADHD also suffer from a variety of comorbid conditions. Brain scans, such as EEG, CT, or MRI, may be done to rule out brain abnormalities that are not consistent with ADHD, and a variety of tests may be given to test IQ and memory and detect learning disabilities and cognitive defects.

Finding Patterns in Childhood Tests

While no single medical, neurological, or attention test reliably identifies ADHD, sometimes doctors can identify patterns across several different tests that point to the presence of the condition.

While the particular combination of tests you take will be determined by your doctor, they will probably include measurements of personality and problem solving styles, current fears and concerns, and intellectual functioning. You may also be asked to take a self-report test in which you answer a series of questions about your symptoms, thoughts, and feelings. Your doctor may also ask a spouse, parent, or close friend to fill out a behavior checklist that describes various behaviors associated with ADHD.

Importance of School and Work Reports

Did you have trouble keeping up in grade school? Were you forced to repeat a grade? Did you do so poorly on college entrance exams that you had to give up on your dreams of becoming a doctor, lawyer, or engineer?

Many adults with ADHD have a history of poor school performance. Your doctor may study your report cards, standardized test scores, reports on teacher-parent meetings, frequent criticism from teachers, and discipline records.

Red Flags on School Records

The three core signs of ADHD are often very easy to spot on past school records. Hyperactivity often shows up on report cards as an inability to sit still, constant fidgeting, or behavior that requires disciplinary action, such as aggression or violence on the playground.

🗒 Fact

Although John managed to graduate from college, his constant "brain fog" forced him to give up his lifelong dream of becoming a scientist. After reviewing John's grade school report cards, John's doctor noticed similar patterns that suggested ADHD and put John on stimulant drugs and therapy. John's brain fog vanished in three months, and he's now studying to become a chemist.

Signs of impulsivity might include cheating on tests or frequent truancy. Low grades, complaints of boredom, or an inability to focus could be signs of childhood inattention.

Studies show that adolescents with ADHD tend to exhibit many of the same inappropriate behavior patterns at school. The developmental histories of adolescents with diagnosed or undiagnosed ADHD are likely to show some of the following aspects:

- Involvement in physically dangerous activities without consideration of possible consequences
- Defiance of the authority of teachers and principals
- Low self-esteem, manifested by putting themselves down, having poor personal care and posture, and communicating negative comments about themselves and others
- Difficulty using unstructured time
- Tendency to lose things needed to complete a task at school
- Tendency to stare off into space
- Tendency to show off, brag, or demand attention as the class clown
- Inability to read nonverbal cues and body language of classmates and teachers
- Displayed sloppy or illegible handwriting
- Tendency to give inappropriate responses in class and to blurt things out

Work-Related Red Flags

Adults with ADHD often experience career difficulties. Problems with concentration and task completion that affect school performance continue to be problems in a job setting. Individuals with adult ADHD tend to have trouble going through established channels and following proper procedure.

Adults with ADHD also don't perform well with rigid authority and may frequently express anger at job requirements or their supervisor. Whatever the reason, adults with ADHD tend to have fewer occupational achievements.

They tend to change employers frequently and may simply quit out of boredom. Poor job performance, inattention, organizational problems, and/or relationship difficulties may also cause frequent job loss. Frequent job changes and poor job performance may leave the finances of many ADHD adults in disarray.

Relationships and Lifestyle Issues

When it comes to their relationships with others, people with adult ADHD often operate at one of two extremes. They may be withdrawn, antisocial, and hermit-like, preferring to spend time alone. Or they may be so extroverted that being alone for even a brief period of time is painful for them. Adults with ADHD at either extreme often find it difficult to make and keep healthy, lasting relationships.

Essential

Adults with ADHD tend to be lonely, isolated, and suffer a high rate of separation and divorce because their erratic and impulsive behavior often alienates friends and family members. This includes blurting out inappropriate comments, flying off the handle, or acting in hostile or aggressive ways.

By interviewing you and your parents, family members, teachers, colleagues, and friends, your physician can get a pretty good sense of your ability to develop and maintain meaningful relationships. This can be helpful in identifying behavior that may cause people to withdraw.

Socioeconomic Clues

Unfortunately, adults with ADHD often have a lower socioeconomic status and less money than other adults, for a variety of factors. Your physician will examine your job records, performance reviews, and salary history to find indications of adult ADHD.

Adults with ADHD typically have higher rates of driving violations, traffic accidents, suspended licenses, drug and alcohol abuse, and psychological maladjustments.

Evaluating Sleep Habits

Your physician will probably also ask you about your sleep habits. Many adults with ADHD have difficulty falling asleep because of anxiety, depression, and racing thoughts. New studies show that various biological factors may also be at play.

According to research published in the journal *SLEEP*, children with ADHD may be chronically sleep deprived and have abnormal REM sleep—factors that could explain or contribute to some hallmark symptoms of ADHD, including erratic behavior, inability to pay attention or focus, hyperactivity, and depression. Children in the study had an average REM sleep time that was significantly reduced by sixteen minutes. While REM is considered the dream stage of sleep, it's not clear why this sleep stage is important. Some researchers theorize it may have something to do with how our brains process information. Scientists hope to examine other factors, including circadian rhythm or changes in brain chemicals like dopamine and norepinephrine (which also play a role in sleep, attention, and arousal) that may link ADHD and sleep.

Examining Eating Habits

Your doctor is likely to ask you about your eating habits, including whether you eat a balanced diet. Studies show that ADHD-like problems can be caused by malnutrition or improper diet, B-vitamin deficiency, and iron deficiency.

Self-Medicating ADHD with Food

Research shows that adults with ADHD may be more likely than others to use food to decrease emotional, physical, and spiritual pain. Unfortunately, the "fix" is usually temporary, but the damaging physical and psychological side effects may take years to heal.

Most "binge" foods preferred by adults with ADHD are packed with sugar and carbohydrates. PET scans showed that ADHD brains were slower to absorb glucose and had a cerebral glucose metabolism that was eight times slower than normal adults.

The Serotonin Connection

Some studies show that adults with ADHD have low levels of serotonin, which may contribute to their feelings of anxiousness, depression, and irritability.

Because foods high in sugar and carbohydrates temporarily raise serotonin levels and relieve those feelings, adults with ADHD may binge on junk food. Adults with ADHD are often prescribed antidepressant medications to elevate serotonin levels, alleviate symptoms of depression, and help improve impulse control.

Eating Disorders and Adult ADHD

If you have adult ADHD, you may also have an increased risk of developing eating disorders. Compulsive overeaters can't control how much they eat. Instead of using food to satisfy their hunger, they eat too many foods high in sugars, carbohydrates, and salt to alter their feelings. Binge eaters are compulsive eaters who not only overeat to feed their feelings, but binge because it gives their lives a sense of excitement and risk. They become obsessed with figuring out where and when to quickly consume large amounts of food so others won't discover them.

Fact

Binge eating followed by purging is called bulimia. In addition to the stimulation, excitement, and rush provided by compulsive eating and bingeing, bulimics report feelings of release, calmness, and euphoria after vomiting. Unfortunately, these feelings are short-lived, and many bulimics repeat the process over and over again to get relief.

Anorexia nervosa, or self-starvation, is also characterized by loss of control—in this case, the ability to think about food in a normal way and eat in a healthy way. Obsessed with thoughts of food, body image, and diet, anorexics may also use laxatives, diuretics, enemas, and compulsive exercise to maintain their distorted image of thinness. Because self-starvation curtails hyperactivity, adults with ADHD may starve themselves in an effort to reduce ADHD symptoms, or they may over-focus on food-related thoughts and behaviors to calm their chaotic minds.

Unfortunately, eating disorders can rob the adult ADHD brain of the nutrients it needs to function and may result in even higher levels of distraction. If you have adult ADHD and you're also struggling with eating disorders, it's important to diagnose and treat both conditions.

Language Disorders and Attention Deficit Hyperactivity Disorder

Your doctor will investigate your childhood history for signs of learning disabilities that often accompany childhood ADHD because the illness is sometimes mistaken for a learning disability.

Most children with ADHD can learn in school without special assistance, even though they may be easily distracted or have trouble sitting still in class. Children with both ADHD and learning disabilities, however, tend to have more severe learning problems than children without ADHD.

ADHD and Learning Styles

Students with ADHD are likely to have trouble listening, sitting still, focusing for extended periods of time, and having good reading and oral language skills. ADHD children are also more likely to have language processing difficulties in a wide variety of areas, including:

- **Syntax.** May have difficulty using and/or comprehending the grammatical and structural components of sentences.
- **Semantics.** May have difficulty comprehending written and spoken language, poor vocabulary, problems finding words, and difficulty using context in reading comprehension.
- **Pragmatics.** May not be able to use language to interact with others socially or to acquire information, express feelings, or conduct a conversation with people of different ages.
- **Metalinguistics.** May not be able to understand and use humor, multiple meanings, ambiguity, and figurative language. May struggle to divide words into syllables and sounds.

Auditory Processing Problems

Children with ADHD may also have auditory processing problems that can make it very difficult for them to follow directions, get information from reading, or listen. They may also have problems with metacognition, or the ability to know what they know and to understand what they need to know in order to learn effectively. Students with difficulties in this area cannot easily deal with the strategies involved in problem solving.

Because ADHD children with language problems can have auditory processing difficulties, your doctor may ask you if you ever had trouble in the following areas:

❑ Problems with remembering information you heard in the short-term
❑ Trouble following instructions
❑ Requiring more time than normal to process written and spoken language
❑ Difficulties listening in environments with noise distractions
❑ Being unable to grasp main ideas or details when someone is talking
❑ Poor writing skills
❑ Inability to engage in classroom discussions
❑ Engaging in tangential narratives and conversations
❑ Difficulty finding the right words in speaking situations
❑ Problems with inferred meaning, or an inability to look beyond the obvious

Children with language and speech disorders are reported to be more likely to have problems with reading, writing, and under-achievement in school. Some research also suggests that disorders of speech and language may increase the risk of having lower IQ scores. The deficits reflected in those scores may continue into adulthood. Chronic problems with speech or language have been shown to increase the likelihood of behavioral problems in children and adults. Research has also suggested that children who have problems with the rules for producing sounds may have lower-skilled employment than siblings who do not have these problems.

Pregnancy and ADHD

Your doctor may study any problems your mother may have had during pregnancy and delivery. If your mother is still living, your physician will probably want to talk to her directly. If she is deceased or not available and you suspect she may have had problems, he may interview you and other family members to try to determine if this was the case.

Anxiety in Pregnancy and Childhood ADHD

Your physician may interview you and/or your parents to find out if your mother experienced significant stress at any time during her pregnancy with you. New research shows that mothers who experience strong anxiety early in pregnancy may increase their child's susceptibility to ADHD years later. In fact, the link between maternal angst and stress and the development of ADHD is stronger than any other predictor of behavioral problems during childhood, including maternal smoking during pregnancy, low birth weight, and a mother's current stress.

The study, which was reported in the journal *Child Development*, showed that maternal anxiety between the twelfth and twenty-second weeks of pregnancy were strongly linked to ADHD. The findings support the controversial hypothesis of fetal programming, a theory that suggests that exposures in the womb play a critical role in predisposing people to a host of diseases and emotional disorders later in life. According to the theory, at certain points during pregnancy environmental exposures to the fetus significantly influence brain development, which, in turn, can impact future health. Other well-publicized research showed that diabetes, heart disease, and obesity are also linked to environmental exposures in the womb.

Maternal Smoking and Childhood ADHD

Your physician may also ask you or your parents if your mother smoked while she was pregnant with you. Recent studies published in *Biological Psychiatry* showed genetic factors combined with prenatal cigarette smoke exposure caused a substantial risk in more serious types of ADHD. In other words, if your mother had adult ADHD and was also a smoker, it may have greatly increased your odds of developing a severe form of childhood ADHD.

Maternal Alcohol Levels and ADHD

Research shows that fetal alcohol syndrome (FAS), or the damage done to children's brains and bodies when their mothers drink heavily during pregnancy, is the leading form of mental retardation today.

In a milder form of prenatal alcohol impairment called fetal alcohol effects (FAE), children often don't look disabled but exhibit a wide range of behavior problems that look much like ADHD and include hyperactivity, attention problems, learning disorders, and ethical problems such as stealing, lying, and cheating. Children with FAE also tend to score in the low-normal or normal ranges on intelligences tests.

ADHD Medications During Pregnancy That Impact ADHD

Although no studies of ADHD management during pregnancy have been conducted, most doctors recommend pregnant women replace stimulant medications with nonpharmacologic approaches.

Searching for Environmental Factors

Make sure your doctor is aware of any environmental toxins you may have been exposed to as a child. Allergies and sensitivities to food and the environment can affect behavior in children, and exposure to toxins can cause hyperactivity, attention deficits, irritability, and learning problems.

The Link Between Toxic Culprits and ADHD

Children are more vulnerable than adults to such toxins as pesticides, gasoline fumes, herbicides, disinfectants, furniture polishes, air fresheners, and/or dust-laden homes. Research shows that mild to high lead levels, even in the absence of clinical lead poisoning, is the leading cause of toxin-induced hyperactivity. Studies show that children with even mildly elevated lead levels have attention deficits, lower IQs, and poor school performance.

Some experts believe that mercury is a neurological poison that may cause many of the symptoms of ADHD, including hyperactivity and poor concentration, although this is quite controversial. These experts believe that mercury amalgam dental fillings that disintegrate when children grind their teeth may release high levels of mercury into the body, and eating large amounts of cold-water fish such as tuna and salmon may also lead to mercury poisoning. Toxic levels of carbon monoxide emitted by gas heaters and other gas appliances such as fireplaces, dryers, and water heaters, can also have ADHD-like side effects in children.

CHAPTER 8

Choosing the Right Treatment

Alleviating adult ADHD symptoms is a top priority of treatment, but the overall goal is to help you function more efficiently, improve your quality of life, and help you cope with the demands of everyday life. Treating adult ADHD is never a one-size-fits all situation, and there are few—if any—cookie-cutter treatment plans. The most effective treatment plans usually include three different types of modalities, including biological, psychological, and behavioral/social interventions. For a comprehensive look at specific treatments, see Chapters 9–13.

Overview of Biological Treatments

Biological treatments alter the way your brain functions. Biological changes can occur as a result of many different factors, including medications and therapies.

Stimulant Medications to Treat Adult ADHD

Psychostimulants continue to be first-line medications for the treatment of ADHD in adults. The most commonly used stimulants are regulated as Schedule II drugs by the Drug Enforcement Administration because they have a potential for abuse when not used as prescribed by a medical professional.

Nonstimulant Medications

In the past, non–stimulant medications were generally considered second-line medications and were limited to people who could not tolerate stimulant medications, did not respond to them, or were not able to use them because of substance abuse issues or coexisting psychiatric conditions.

All that changed in 2003, when the nonstimulant drug Strattera arrived on the market. Strattera is the only nonstimulant medication to be approved by the Food and Drug Administration (FDA) for the treatment of ADHD and the first medication of any kind specifically approved for the treatment of ADHD in adults. Because Strattera doesn't have the abuse potential of stimulants, and because it isn't a controlled Schedule II drug, it can be prescribed with refills and over the phone. However, it may not be as effective as stimulant mediation.

Other Types of Medication

If neither stimulant drugs nor Strattera work for you, your physician may prescribe antidepressants. Research shows that SSRIs have a positive effect on the core symptoms of ADHD. Tricyclic Antidepressants (TCAs) may also help with core symptoms such as anxiety and depression. If neither of these is helpful, your doctor may prescribe bupropion, also known as Wellbutrin (for depression) or Zyban (for smoking cessation). Bupropion is an antidepressant and anti-smoking medication that also seems to elevate mood and relieve depression.

Other drugs that may be prescribed on an "off-label" basis to help with adult ADHD symptoms include blood pressure medications, antihypertensive agents, and wake-promoting agents used to control narcolepsy. For a comprehensive look at medications used to treat adult ADHD, including the pros, cons, and side effects associated with them, see Chapter 9.

Psychological Treatments for Adult ADHD

Psychological treatments for adult ADHD include treatments that help you cope with the secondary symptoms of the disorder—in other words, the feelings of anger, frustration, hostility, impatience, low self-esteem, hopelessness, helplessness, guilt, blame, and fear that arise from the primary symptoms of adult ADHD.

Some types of psychological treatment help you see and understand why you feel the way you do. Others help you find ways to cope with the effects of living with the symptoms of adult ADHD, or modify your behavior and thoughts using conditioning and association.

Changing Your Attitudes Through Counseling and Psychotherapy

Counseling and psychotherapy can involve standard talk therapy, treatments that teach you how to change the way you think and act, and therapies that enable you to vent pent-up feelings. While counseling and psychotherapy can't eliminate the symptoms of adult ADHD, it can help you develop strategies to better cope with your symptoms.

For instance, counseling can help you accept the fact that you have the disorder as well as the problems that accompany it. Once you accept you have the disorder, you can look for ways to adjust your personal and work life so things run more smoothly. Counseling can also help remove any guilt or shame you may be feeling about your symptoms by helping you better understand their neurobiological origins.

Adjusting Your Behavior Through Cognitive-Behavioral Therapy

In cognitive-behavioral therapy, you learn to adjust your behavior by identifying patterns of thought and behavior and using various techniques to modify them. This short-term therapy has been shown to work as well as antidepressants for treating mild to moderate depression.

Patients identify and reduce the frequent, intense negative thoughts that lead to their depression, and then replace these self-destructive thoughts with more realistic and constructive thoughts. This relieves distress and helps motivate them toward positive action.

In this type of therapy, your therapist may ask you to write down what you were thinking before, during, and after episodes of negative behavior, and record how often you engage in negative behavior. This allows you to get a better picture of why, how, when, and how frequently negative thoughts and behavior interrupt your life.

Essential

Keeping records of the way you feel, think, and act can help you find patterns between them so you can look for ways to modify them. In the final steps of cognitive-behavioral counseling, you replace negative thoughts with positive ones. You also change your behavior using conditioning principles.

Your therapist may also ask you to rate the intensity of emotions that accompany your thoughts so you can see how strongly you feel about a certain behavior or how motivated you feel to act in that particular way.

Monitoring Your Thoughts with Awareness Training

In awareness training, you work with a counselor to develop increased awareness of yourself and your environment. The goal of awareness training is to become more in tune with how you think, feel, and act. Tapping into this "streaming" information can help you consciously change the way you behave.

Psychoeducational Counseling

This type of counseling emphasizes understanding adult ADHD and finding new skills for living with it. Your counselor will likely discuss topics like adult ADHD symptoms, various treatments and medications, alternative treatments, coexisting conditions, support groups, special assistance at work or school, disability issues, and insurance concerns.

Sharing Experiences Through Group Therapy

In group therapy, people with similar problems or issues meet regularly as a group with a therapist to discuss problems, share experiences, and find solutions.

Adults with ADHD typically have poor planning and organizational skills and can be difficult to live and work with. In family counseling, the entire family meets with a therapist to better understand family members with ADHD and to find family solutions for creating harmony at home and supporting family members with the disorder. Couples where one or both partners have adult ADHD may find group therapy helpful in working out issues stemming from adult ADHD symptoms such as forgetfulness, carelessness, lack of patience, and having a short temper.

Developing Specific Skills Through Training

Training is a form of counseling that helps you develop or improve specific skills you may need in a variety of situations, both at home and in your job. It is also a valuable type of therapy for adults with ADHD who aren't comfortable with approaches used in standard talk therapy.

Instead of examining your emotions and what motivates you to think and behave in a certain way, training helps you focus exclusively on improving or developing the concrete skills you need to function in a more efficient way.

Many people discover that developing new skills helps so much that they begin to think and act in a more positive and life-affirming way. As a result, they often find themselves functioning more efficiently and appropriately at work, at school, and in social settings.

Neurofeedback Therapies

Neurofeedback, which is also called EEG-biofeedback or neurotherapy, works on the assumption that you can improve the symptoms of adult ADHD by changing the level of activity in the brain. During neurofeedback, you're hooked up to an EEG machine and electrodes are attached to your scalp that (painlessly) deliver a baseline report of your brain activity. Your baseline report is then compared against a databank of "normal" baselines to measure differences. You repeatedly perform learning exercises aimed at improving areas where your brain function is weak.

Experimental Therapies

Many adults with ADHD use balancing therapies like visits to the chiropractor, osteopathy, yoga, transcendental meditation, acupuncture, acupressure, and homeopathy, to reduce stress, slow racing thoughts, and experience feelings of calm and tranquility.

Experimental therapies include sensory integration therapies, which may help you process stimuli more effectively; auditory integration training, which could assist with the processing of auditory stimuli; and vision therapy, which may help improve visual processing.

Although the results of rebalancing and experimental therapies have not been scientifically documented, many adults with ADHD find them extremely helpful in alleviating symptoms. Although these therapies are not usually prescribed in lieu of other biological treatments, they may be useful complements to your treatment program.

The Benefits of Diet and Exercise

Engaging in regular aerobic exercise and eating a diet low in simple carbohydrates and high in dietary protein are two nonmedical ways that may help keep adult ADHD symptoms at bay.

The Staying Power of Protein and Whole Grains

A diet high in protein prevents your blood sugar levels from spiking, which causes hyperactivity and nervousness, or from crashing, which can leave you feeling tired, lethargic, irritable, and depressed. Dietary protein also triggers the synthesis of neurotransmitters like dopamine and norepinephrine, which deliver a boost of energy, as well as neurotransmitters like serotonin, which help you relax and fall asleep. Eating several servings of whole grains a day also helps prevent wild fluctuations in blood sugars that can either make you feel wired and/or exhausted.

Essential

Several studies show that adults with ADHD who take fish oil and omega-3 supplements enjoy an even bigger boost in mental focus than people who don't suffer from the disorder. Most people begin to see mental benefits six weeks after taking the supplements.

While the ADHD diet will probably not eliminate all your adult ADHD symptoms, it could help prevent major swings in mood and behavior, ward off hunger (which could cause irritability, grumpiness, and lethargy), and prevent nutritional deficiencies. The diet could also boost your energy, help you relax and sleep, and make it easier to lose weight and keep it off.

The Aerobics Advantage

If you have adult ADHD and you're also a longtime couch potato, your physician may suggest that you embark on a regular program of aerobic exercise such as walking, hiking, or cycling. Although aerobic exercise will firm up flab and tone your muscles, it's equally healthy for your brain. Just a half hour of exercise four times a week increases your brain's levels of dopamine, norepineprhine, and serotonin—three neurotransmitters that not only improve your focus and attention, but enhance feelings of well-being.

Exercise is also the ultimate empowerment tool, reducing feelings of helplessness and hopelessness and making you feel like you can conquer your adult ADHD symptoms. Exercise that involves a high degree of technical expertise and hand-eye coordination, such as rock climbing, skating, ballet, gymnastics, and white-water canoeing, also help strengthen parts of your brain responsible for controlling fine motor skills, balance, timing, and sequencing. They encourage your brain to correct mistakes and anticipate the next move.

Fact

When you're literally between a rock and a hard place, everything else in the world tends to vanish. That's why high-octane sports like climbing, canoeing, and mountain biking can improve your ability to pinpoint focus, pay attention, and block out extraneous and potentially dangerous distractions.

Because exercise also releases serotonin, the "feel-good" hormone, you're also likely to feel less stressed, more centered, and more at peace with the world. Exercise in the morning to get yourself moving and in the late afternoon to improve the quality of your sleep.

Building Social Skills

Many adults with ADHD manifest their symptoms in a variety of socially unacceptable ways. They may be rude or impatient with others, butt into conversations or lines without being invited, or blurt out inappropriate comments. The disorder may also cause them to be chronically late, forgetful, sloppy, or careless—symptoms that others may mistake for a lack of caring or interest.

Many adults also have negative behavior patterns that alienate friends, colleagues, and family members. As a result, many adults with ADHD feel like social outcasts or misfits, and may be very isolated and lonely. Social skills can also help adults with the disorder rebuild the social niceties they need.

Benefits of a Multi-Treatment Approach

Most experts agree that the best way to tackle adult ADHD is through a multi-treatment approach that combines medication, psychotherapy, and social skills. While medication is generally regarded as the first line of defense in treating adult ADHD, experts concur that "pills do not substitute for skills."

While medication can certainly level the neurobiological playing field and allow adults with ADHD to learn and develop the skills they need to succeed, it won't help them improve on problems organizing, managing time, prioritizing, and using cognitive aids. For this reason, medication should be just one part of an adult's treatment plan. Some people know what to do but have not been able to do it because their symptoms have so severely impacted their ability to organize and plan. Once their symptoms diminish, they can put the effective behaviors they already know to work.

Different Strokes for Different Folks

The best treatment plan is usually a team approach that combines several different treatment modalities and is customized for each person. One person may find that medication works best in combination with diet, exercise, stress management, and counseling. Another person may prefer a nonchemical alternative route that combines counseling, stress reduction, vitamin and herbal therapy, and coaches. Still others may prefer a blended approach that combines traditional medicine with some alternative therapies like yoga and meditation.

The Saving Grace of Variety

Using a variety of different treatments also increases the chances that you'll enjoy more continuous relief from symptoms in the event one or more of your treatments are no longer effective, stop working on a temporary basis, or you need to stop one or more treatments for a variety of reasons.

Tools for Charting Your Progress

Here are five easy ways to stay on top of things.

- Invest in a day calendar that has a large enough space for each day so you can keep track of various and sundry details. Break it up into home, work, and personal time, and put notes, tips, and reminders under each category. Use it to jot down everything from doctor's appointments and important phone numbers to reactions to medications, stress-busting strategies, and work deadlines.
- Use a diary as a companion to your day calendar. Keeping a diary or day journal is a great way to relieve stress, rant and rave, and record private thoughts and emotions you may not be comfortable discussing with others. Once you write something down, it's not only off your chest, but it also helps you look at the thoughts or actions more objectively. Because remembering things may not be your forte, a journal can also help you stay on top of important dates and occasions.

- Create a medications journal to record when, why, and how your adult ADHD symptoms wax and wane, your reactions to new medications or changes in dosages, how various treatments make you feel, and which treatments work and don't work for you. This will help you take medications as directed. Missing a dose or taking two doses at once to catch up on missed doses can have negative consequences for you and others. If you are noticing side effects or other problems, speak to your health care provider as soon as possible.

- Make a daily "mood" chart with categories for exercise, hours of sunshine, sleep, nutrition, and stress relief. Rate your mood on a scale of one to ten, then engage in activities designed to increase relaxation and happiness, giving yourself a check for 30 minutes of daily exercise, 30 minutes of sunshine, seven hours of sleep, a healthy diet low in sugar and carbohydrates, and stress-reducing activities like yoga or meditation.

- Become a list master. Make lists of daily tasks you need to achieve, and then strike them off as you complete them to achieve a sense of accomplishment. Create lists for routine tasks like grocery shopping and errands so you don't arrive home from shopping with only half of the things you needed. If you have a busy day at work, list everything you need to do in chronological order. This will help you correct scheduling errors before they occur. If you're seeing your doctor, make a list of questions to ask him as well as lists of other relevant information, such as medications you take and their dosages.

Self-Education Tips and Strategies

The more you know about adult ADHD and the more tools and strategies you have at your disposal, the better you'll be able to manage the various mental, emotional, physical, and lifestyle challenges, setbacks, and detours arising from living with the disorder. Here are ten easy things you can do yourself to minimize the symptoms of adult ADHD.

1. Get to the root of things. If you or someone you love has been feeling out of sorts or showing signs of depression for two weeks or longer, it's important to get to the root of the problem. Adults with ADHD can suffer from primary or secondary depression, or both.

   While primary depression is largely inherited and not triggered by life problems like job loss or relationship problems, secondary depression usually results from the accumulated frustrations and disappointments of living with undiagnosed or untreated adult ADHD. Don't be afraid to ask for help if you feel like your life is spiraling out of control because of disruptive thoughts or behaviors.

2. Find ways to minimize distractions. If you have adult ADHD, you already have trouble maintaining focus and shifting attention to something else when it's necessary. Find ways to reduce distractions. To avoid being distracted by loud music or television, turn down the volume, turn it off altogether, or use ear plugs or white noise machines to block or camouflage the noise. If you work in a noisy, distracting environment, ask your boss if you can move to an office or cubicle that's quieter and has fewer distractions. Find or create a quiet corner at home where you can catch up on household bills and problems without being interrupted by children or spouses. If you live in a noisy city, drown out traffic and street noise with a white-noise machine that emits soothing nature sounds, such as falling rain, waterfalls, crashing waves, thunderstorms, and chirping crickets.

3. Improve your quality of life. Don't assume that having adult ADHD means you have to put up with depression

and anxiety. If you're on ADHD medication and still suffer from mild to moderate depression, ask your doctor about prescribing an antidepressant. Antidepressants boost levels of the neurotransmitters serotonin and norepinephrine, and will help you maintain feelings of well-being and happiness.

4. Easy does it on carbohydrates and caffeine. Adults with ADHD often resort to high-carbohydrate snacks or frequent consumption of caffeine to elevate their mood or increase alertness and energy. Unfortunately, the "fix" doesn't last long. Overdoing carbohydrates can lead to weight gain and fatigue, while too much caffeine can make you feel nervous and jittery and lead to insomnia. It's better to stick with a low-carb, protein-rich breakfast and to snack on fruits and nuts instead of sugar and starch.

   To maintain a healthy low-carb, high-protein diet, invest in cookbooks like *The South Beach Diet* or *The Zone*, both of which have low-carb meal plans, recipes, and lists of good versus bad carbohydrates. To keep track of how much coffee you drink, keep a small chart by the coffee pot, or make a deal with yourself to make just one small pot of coffee each morning, and then switch to noncaffeinated teas in the afternoon and evening, particularly if you are having trouble sleeping.

5. Ward off the blues by creating an "anti-boredom" closet. Studies show that many adults with ADHD get depressed when they have nothing to do. Adults with ADHD sometimes have more nervous energy than others, and this hyperactivity needs to have an outlet of some sort. To prevent idleness or boredom from tanking your mood, create an anti-boredom closet and stock it with books, games, arts or crafts supplies, sports equipment, and projects that absolutely fascinate you but you can't find time for in your

everyday life. The next time you find yourself facing an unexpected block of free time, instead of fretting or panicking, head to your anti-boredom closet and find something to capture your imagination.

6. Chart your sleep. Many adults with ADHD have trouble falling asleep, which can worsen symptoms of inattention and focus. To get a handle on your sleep habits, keep a chart of when you go to bed every night, how much sleep you get, how often you get up at night, and when you wake up in the morning. For a good night's sleep, go to bed at the same time every night; get up at the same time every morning; avoid exercise, TV, and other stimulating activities for at least an hour before going to bed; and limit caffeine consumption to the morning hours. You may also want to avoid eating a heavy meal right before bedtime. If you have trouble falling asleep, or you find yourself waking up several times during the night, you may want to ask your physician about sleep medications. Remember that worrying about whether you will be able to sleep is in itself a contributor to insomnia.

7. Zone in on stress triggers. If you feel overwhelmed by stress, don't shut down—write it down. List the biggest stresses in your day on a piece of paper, and then start looking for ways to reduce or eliminate them. If you can't eliminate the source of stress from your life, such as a hectoring boss or demanding child, try to change the way you react to it.

   Charting your progress can also help you move toward action. A few tools and strategies can go a long way toward keeping your treatment progress and everyday life in order.

8. Find new ways to calm your body and soul. Sit quietly with your eyes closed and focus on your breathing to meditate. Each time you exhale, silently repeat a one-syllable word—"one" or "peace" or "ohm." Experts suggest

trying for a few minutes or even for a few seconds every time you find yourself in a panic or funk. If you can't sit still long enough to meditate, try walking meditation or tai chi, a type of "moving" yoga.

9. Keep a lid on impulsive behavior. If you have a tendency to do things you later regret, such as interrupting or getting angry at others, keep your impulses in check by counting to ten while breathing slowly instead of acting out. You'll be surprised to find that most of your impulses evaporate as quickly as they appeared.

10. Find constructive outlets for excess energy. People with ADHD sometimes seem to have more nervous energy than others, and this hyperactivity needs to have an outlet of some sort. A hobby or other pastime can be helpful.

These ten strategies are just a starter list. Brainstorm for additional ways to keep adult ADHD symptoms in check with members of your support group, or get an "adult ADHD buddy" and develop strategies together to solve problems as they arise. Experts' estimates suggest that depression is 2.7 times more prevalent in ADHD adults than it is in the general adult population. By using these remedies and strategies, you can fend off depression and be in the best physical shape of your life.

The Power of Support Groups

You already know how and why adult ADHD can leave you feeling lonely and isolated. One of the easiest and fastest ways to make connections with other adults struggling with ADHD is to join a support group in your area.

As well as providing a way to make new friends, share your experiences and problems, and offer moral support, your support group can also keep you informed on the best medical resources, special services, disability experts, and colleges and universities that cater to adults with ADHD. To find a support group near you, check with local colleges, universities, churches and synagogues, community hospitals and clinics, senior citizen centers, and the local chapter of CHADD, an organization for children and adults with ADHD. If you can't find a support group in your community, you can always start one of your own.

Keeping Up with ADHD Research

Research on adult ADHD is ongoing. Nearly every month scientists uncover new findings about possible causes of the disorder and new treatments to help alleviate symptoms. To stay up with the latest and greatest research findings, check out professional magazines in the field of psychology and psychiatry.

Start with *The Journal of Neuropsychiatry and Clinical Neurosciences*, the *American Journal of Psychiatry*, and *Neuropsychology*. You can also find breaking news on the latest studies and research in consumer magazines like *Science* and *Psychology*, newspapers like *The Wall Street Journal*, and in hundreds of other publications.

Medical search databases are another way to find a wealth of information on adult ADHD research and studies. By simply typing in "adult ADHD," you'll get instant access to articles and abstracts from a variety of magazines and newspapers.

Some of the best medical website databases include the U.S. National Library of Medicine (*www.nlm.nih.gov*), with links to Medline; and Medscape (*www.medscape.com*).

CHAPTER 9

Treating with Medication

Medications for adult ADHD affect the neurotransmitters in your brain responsible for attention and motivation. While stimulant drugs have long been considered the first line of defense in treating the disorder and are still widely regarded as the most effective, they are by no means the only type of medication. Many nonstimulant drugs, including antidepressants, anticonvulsants, waking agents, and even estrogen have proven beneficial. Strattera, a relatively new nonstimulant drug that's the only medication approved by the FDA specifically for adult ADHD, is showing great promise in treating the disorder.

National Institutes of Health Landmark Study

Adult ADHD and depression often go hand-in-hand, and a multi-treatment approach often works best to alleviate symptoms of the disorder. Results of a 2006 landmark study funded by the NIH showed that using a variety of antidepressants may also help relieve depression in adults.

In the study, one out of three people suffering from chronic depression found relief from symptoms after adding a second medication, and one in four became symptom-free after switching to a different antidepressant. The medications included sertraline (Zoloft), bupropion-SR (Wellbutrin), and venlaxafine-XR (Effexor), three different types of antidepressants.

Essential

To date, no psychostimulants routinely prescribed for adult ADHD have been approved by the FDA specifically for the treatment of the disorder. For this reason, these drugs are often prescribed "off label," or used for reasons other than the standard prescribed use.

The research also showed that the best course of action if your first treatment or medication isn't successful is to work with your physician to change or add another medication until you find a combination that works. Studies have shown that stimulant medication is a safe, long-term solution for adult ADHD.

Challenges in Medicating Adults with ADHD

Research funded by NIMH indicates that medication is most effective when treatment is routinely monitored by a physician. Adults may also benefit from a change in dose or scheduling. Long-acting medications that are taken once a day, rather than in multiple doses, seem to work best for most adults.

Short duration stimulants may wear off quickly. Since many adult patients have problems with forgetfulness, taking multiple doses during the day can leave them unprotected if they forget to take the second and third doses. Adults who are tempted to take stimulants at night to help them calm down may wind up feeling so relaxed they can't focus on household chores, homework, completing projects for work, paying bills, or even driving.

The Problem with Substance Abuse

Research shows that 60 to 80 percent of adults with ADHD experience a dramatic reduction of symptoms after taking stimulant drugs. While using stimulants to treat adult ADHD may seem paradoxical, studies show mild stimulants have a dramatic calming effect on the brains and nerves of adults with ADHD and also reduce the incidence of substance abuse among treated adults. However, because many adults with ADHD have a history of substance abuse, and because stimulant drugs are schedule II controlled substances, some believe there's a chance they may be tempted to use their ADHD medication for recreational purposes.

Fact

Research shows that adults with ADHD being treated with stimulants have a lower incidence of substance abuse that other adults, and are also less likely to self-medicate with illegal substances than adults with undiagnosed adult ADHD. Recent studies showed that the majority of adults taking Ritalin gradually lower their dose of stimulants across time rather than increasing the dose.

For people with a recent history of substance use but no current use, deciding to use stimulant medication should be dealt with on a case-by-case basis. Certain extended release preparations are less likely to be abused. One example is Concerta, which can't be crushed and used other than as prescribed orally.

In general, medications with a gradual onset of effect and long durations of effect are likely to work most smoothly, avoiding emotional ups and downs. These are also the best formulations for people with a history of substance abuse because they avoid the "hit" and "buzz" of recreational stimulants.

Vyvanse, a new medication for adult ADHD, is a "pro-drug." After you ingest the medication, the body converts it to a stimulant, which lessens the potential for abuse.

Differences in Treating Children and Adults

While many of the medications are the same as those used for children and adolescents, there are several general differences to consider. Although adults are generally larger than children, they may need less medication per pound of body weight because the drug may remain in their system longer if they don't have healthy liver and kidney function.

In addition, adults are more likely to be taking medications for other conditions, some of which may interact with ADHD drugs and interfere with their potency. Many medications taken by adults for coexisting conditions may also cause lethargy, anxiety, and insomnia or exacerbate adult ADHD symptoms.

The Practice of Polypharmacy

Polypharmacy, or prescribing several psychiatric medications at the same time, is often used to treat coexisting conditions in adults with ADHD. For instance, if an adult has ADHD as well as clinical anxiety, she may need to take medication for both conditions. If done in the right way, polypharmacy can result in a simultaneous reduction of symptoms for both conditions. But if medications are prescribed without taking into account their various side effects, a patient could suffer serious medical consequences or even experience an increase in symptoms.

Most Commonly Prescribed Drugs to Treat Adult ADHD

Over the past fifteen years, the medication options for treating adult ADHD have greatly expanded. Today, the most popular medications for treating the disease include stimulant drugs and a wide variety of nonstimulant drugs in various drug categories.

Despite the growing number of medication options, stimulant medications, including methylphenidate (such as Ritalin), and dextroamphetamine compounds (such as Dextrostat, Dexedrine Spansules, and Adderall) remain the most commonly prescribed drugs for adult ADHD.

Stimulant medications like Ritalin and Adderall remain the most frequently prescribed drugs, but they are no longer the only line of defense for adults with ADHD. Other medications that are sometimes prescribed off-label for adult ADHD include TCAs such as Elavil.

Medications that may be prescribed for comorbid conditions include serotonin selective reuptake inhibitors, such as Prozac and Zoloft, and mood stabilizers. Although no antidepressants have been approved by the FDA for treating adult ADHD, they are often prescribed off-label to alleviate its symptoms.

In 2002, the nonstimulant drug Strattera became the first medication approved by the FDA specifically for the treatment of ADHD in adults. Strattera is not a Class II stimulant, so there is also no abuse potential.

Things to Remember If You're Considering Medication

Drug treatment for adult ADHD requires that you maintain an open line of communication with your physician to ensure you are taking the right drug at the right dose. This can be vital if you suffer adverse side effects and need to take corrective measures or if a drug stops working for you.

Medications are not magic bullets or cures, but part of an overall treatment approach. Because the first medication you try may not be the drug that offers you the most benefits, it's important to pay attention to how medications affect your symptoms and what side effects occur.

Essential

Medication for adult ADHD can help relieve symptoms, but it should not be regarded as a substitute for mastering strategies and healthy lifestyle habits or for the many types of therapies that could help you better cope on a daily basis with the symptoms and challenges presented by the disorder.

Remember to be patient; you and your doctor may need to experiment with various medications before you find the medication, amount, and dosing schedule that works best for you.

The Role of Clinical Trials

Clinical trials are done to isolate distinct symptoms of ADHD in adults as well as to develop new medications and treatments. However, more clinical trials are needed to determine if adult ADHD medications both alleviate symptoms and lead to permanent improvements in executive functions like planning, organizing, and prioritizing.

Focus on Stimulant Drugs

Stimulants come in a variety of forms and brands. Stimulant medications are considered safe when taken under medical supervision. Used as prescribed, they do not make adults with ADHD feel high.

Although the majority—60 to 80 percent—of adults with ADHD enjoy a dramatic decrease in symptoms when taking medication, some only receive a small benefit while others reap none at all. Others suffer from side effects that are so severe that they must go off the drugs.

How Stimulants Work in the Brain

Stimulant medications are believed to directly affect the brain neurotransmitters dopamine and norepinephrine, which are responsible for transmitting messages between different parts of the brain.

Dopamine controls the power of the signals coming into your brain and regulates areas of the brain that control filtering and screening. Norepinephrine controls your level of alertness, clarity, and wakefulness. Both neurotransmitters have an impact on motivation and are also believed to affect attention and behavioral symptoms, although how this works remains unknown.

Alert

Seventy-five percent of adults with ADHD also have co-existing conditions. However, there are no controlled studies on the most effective ways to treat adults with overlapping conditions, so physicians must rely on their previous clinical experience and continual feedback from patients to find a treatment plan that works for each patient.

Generic stimulants are usually inexpensive, although many longer acting stimulants can be quite expensive if your insurance doesn't cover medication costs.

Forms of Stimulant Medication

Stimulant medications come in pills, capsules, liquids, and skin patches. Some medications also come in short-acting, long-acting, or extended release varieties. The active ingredient is the same in each of these varieties, but it is released differently in the body.

Long-acting or extended release forms ("ER" or "XR") often work best for adults who need continuous relief during daytime and evening hours and who may be too forgetful or distracted to remember to take second and third doses. They are also prescribed to people for whom substance abuse is a concern.

The Half-Life of Medication

The half-life of a drug refers to the amount of time it takes a drug to reach 50 percent of its peak effectiveness after you take a dose. The longer the half-life of a drug, the longer it takes for the drug to reach its full effect, and the more important it is to take it on time to maintain a steady level of medication in your bloodstream.

Neglecting to take drugs with a short half-life on time may result in a condition called discontinuation syndrome. Symptoms include irritability, insomnia, dizziness, light-headedness, and flu-like symptoms, and may persist for weeks.

Commonly Prescribed Stimulants

There are many different kinds of stimulant drugs your physician may prescribe. Although they all work in a similar fashion, the differ in how quickly they begin to work, how long they remain in your bloodstream, the degree of relief they provide, and their side effects. Through trial-and-error, you and your physician will be able to determine which medication(s) work best for you.

Methylphenidate

Marketed as Ritalin, Concerta, Metadate, and Focalin, methylphenidate is one of the most widely prescribed drugs for adult ADHD and is available in a wide range of forms. Different brands use different delivery systems to get the medication into your system, and there are also differences among brands in how long the drugs take to reach their half-life and peak, how long they remain in the bloodstream, and their side effects. Methylphenidate is available in a variety of forms, including short-acting, long-acting, and sustained-release.

Dexedrine (D-Amphetamine)

Dexedrine is one of the oldest drugs used to treat adult ADHD and is still considered one of the best. It is offered in both short-acting and sustained-released forms.

Adderall (Salts of D- and L-Amphetamine)

Similar to Dexedrine, this medication is believed to have more impact on norepinephrine than Dexedrine. It is available in short- and long-acting forms.

Vyvanse

This newer medication is similar to Adderall in its chemical composition. It is believed to have less potential for substance abuse than most stimulants because snorting it or injecting it will not cause a user to get high. Before it can become effective, the body must convert it from its oral form to a stimulant form. It may result in a smoother onset and result in less restlessness than Adderall.

Dexoxyn (Methamphetamine)

Biologically identical to the methamphetamine manufactured in illegal drug labs, Dexoxyn has gotten an undeserved bad rap. The legal, prescription form of Dexoxyn is not only one of the most beneficial medications for many adults with ADHD, but one of the least expensive medications.

Cylert (Pemoline)

This medication causes the release of dopamine but not norepinephrine. Because the drug has been associated with liver damage, it is only prescribed after other stimulants have failed. People who take Cylert are generally advised to get regular liver function tests.

Provigil (Modafinil)

Although this drug is approved for the treatment of narcolepsy, research indicates it may have some benefit in adults with ADHD, although the drug does not appear to increase the levels of dopamine and norepinephrine.

Side Effects of Stimulants

The most common adverse reactions in double-blind clinical trails were decreased appetite, headache, dry mouth, nausea, insomnia, anxiety, dizziness, weight loss, and irritability. The most common adverse reactions associated with discontinuation from adult clinical trials were anxiety, irritability, insomnia, and increases in blood pressure. However, it should be noted that most side effects are minor and disappear over time or if the dosage level is lowered.

Dealing with Stimulant-Related Sleep Problems

If you can't fall asleep, ask your doctor about prescribing a lower dose of the medication or a shorter-acting form for use in the afternoon or early evening. You might also ask about taking the medication earlier in the day, or stopping the afternoon or evening dose.

A low dose of certain antidepressants or a blood pressure medication called Clonidine may also help alleviate sleep problems. Maintaining a good sleep schedule is also important, so make sure you go to bed and get up at the same time every day, end the day with relaxing activities, and establish a relaxing sleep environment. Using black-out eye shades, ear plugs, and white-noise machines can help eliminate distractions like bright lights and noise.

Strattera, a Rising Star in Medications

Although nonstimulants like antidepressants and mood stabilizers have been used for years to alleviate symptoms of adult ADHD, few have created the same excitement and buzz as Strattera. The only nonstimulant medication to be approved by the FDA for the treatment of ADHD, Strattera is also the first medication of any sort to be specifically approved by the FDA for the treatment of ADHD in adults.

Strattera works like an antidepressant to strengthen the chemical signal between nerves that use the neurotransmitter norepinephrine to send messages. Unlike SSRIs, Strattera does not impact serotonin levels in the brain.

 Fact

Although research is still ongoing, many scientists believe that Strattera could one day be as widely prescribed and beneficial for treating adult ADHD as stimulant drugs. In long-term studies, two-thirds of adults taking Strattera enjoyed relief from symptoms for longer than thirty-four weeks.

Strattera may be helpful to those who cannot tolerate stimulants, although some patients claim stimulant drugs are more effective in controlling their ADHD symptoms. The medication is taken once a day, although those suffering gastrointestinal upset can take a smaller dose twice a day. Full effects are usually felt within four to six weeks and last all day and sometimes even into the next morning.

Common Side Effects

Common side effects include headache, abdominal pain, nausea, vomiting, weight loss, anxiety, sleepiness and insomnia. Strattera can also interfere with sexual performance. Studies show that Strattera may cause less insomnia, appetite suppression, and weight loss than methylphenidate, but more sleepiness and vomiting.

Nonstimulant Medications

With the exception of Strattera, most other nonstimulant medications are generally considered second-line medications for adult ADHD. They tend to be prescribed for people who either had a bad response to stimulants, couldn't tolerate the side effects, or have co-existing psychiatric conditions that rule out stimulant drugs.

Selective Serotonin Reuptake Inhibitors

Prescribed for depression, anxiety, obsessive-compulsive disorder, and anger and aggression, SSRIs are most useful in alleviating coexisting symptoms of conditions accompanying adult ADHD. They work primarily by eliminating serotonin from the brain's synapses, though they may affect other neurotransmitters to a lesser degree.

Popular SSRIs include Prozac, the oldest SSRI, which has a long half-life but many known drug interactions; Luvox, which is similar to Prozac but has a shorter half-life and fewer drug reactions; Paxil, a short-acting SSRI which may pose problems with dosing and discontinuation syndrome; and Zoloft, another short-acting SSRI that also has an effect on dopamine and may offer some of the benefits of stimulant drugs.

Other SSRIs sometimes prescribed to adults with ADHD include Celexa and Lexapro. Both have longer half-lives than all other SSRIs except Prozac and fewer drug reactions than most SSRIs. Lexapro is often preferred because it is more potent and has fewer side effects.

SSRIs have several side effects, many of which are mild or which affect only a small percentage of people. The most troublesome side effects may include weight gain, drowsiness, irritability, and thinning hair or hair loss.

Serotonin/Norepinephrine Reuptake Inhibitors

These antidepressants impact the levels of both serotonin and norepinephrine, and are useful in treating depression, anxiety, and adult ADHD. However, they generally don't offer the symptom relief of stimulant drugs and are often prescribed when stimulant drugs don't work, or in addition to stimulant drugs.

One widely prescribed drug in this category is Effexor, which seems to stimulate energy as well as lead to a calming feeling. Although there are no controlled studies on the use of Effexor in adults with ADHD, several noncontrolled studies indicate that it may be especially helpful in treating adult ADHD with coexisting depression and/or anxiety. However, side effects of higher doses may increase blood pressure, and sudden discontinuation of Effexor could lead to nausea and vomiting.

Another popular drug in this category is Remeron, which works on serotonin, norepinephrine, and histamine to promote sleep, increase energy, and increase appetite. However, one major side effect is a dramatic increase in appetite and a constant craving for carbohydrates. Remeron also makes many people very drowsy.

Tricyclic Antidepressants

TCAs, the first medications developed to treat depression, work by significantly inhibiting serotonin and norepinephrine reuptake.

TCAs have negligible risk of abuse and are especially beneficial when treating ADHD adults who also have coexisting anxiety and depression. On the downside, it may take several weeks for the drugs to have a full clinical effect, and TCAs generally don't offer the relief of stimulants. Unfortunately, they do have overdose potential and should be monitored. TCAs prescribed for adult ADHD include Elavil, Sinequan, and Nortriptyline, all of which have sedating qualities. Elavil has the strongest sedative, while Nortriptyline has the weakest.

Another TCA, Norpramine, has proven beneficial in adults with ADHD when given in small doses. Anafranil, another TCA, impacts serotonin levels and is often prescribed for ADHD adults also suffering from compulsive disorders.

Side effects of TCAs range from sleepiness and constipation to light-headedness and dry mouth. More serious conditions include cardiac problems and possible death by overdose.

Mono–amine Oxidase Inhibitors (MAOIs)

MAOIs help ADHD by blocking the breakdown of norepinephrine, dopamine, and serotonin. Most frequently prescribed MAOIs include Nardil, Parnate, and Elderpril.

Because there are no controlled studies on the treatment of ADHD in adults with MAOIs and those using MAOIs must adhere to a strict diet to prevent an acute rise in blood pressure or hypertension, MAOIs are usually limited to adults with ADHD who have resisted other forms of treatment. They have also proven beneficial in treating adults with nonimpulsive adult ADHD symptoms and in ADHD adults who have coexisting depression and anxiety.

Anti-Smoking Drugs

Bupropion SR and XL (Wellbutrin) has been used to treat ADHD. Bupropion increases dopamine and norepinephrine levels and is reported to have a moderate response in adults with ADHD, although the effect is not considered as strong as stimulants and may take several weeks to kick in.

A recent controlled study showed that the drug is effective in the treatment of ADHD symptoms in adults. Although the drug is chemically similar to amphetamine, it does not have the same potential for abuse. Drug manufacturers still warn that it should not be used by people with a history of substance abuse, bulimia, or seizure disorders.

Mood Stabilizers and Antihypertensives

Mood stabilizers are prescribed to help modulate irritability and rapid mood shifts. The most widely prescribed mood stabilizers include Lithium, Depakote, Tegretol, and Lamictal.

Antihypertensives are used to decrease hyperactivity and impulsivity in adults with ADHD and may also help relieve insomnia. Drugs commonly prescribed for adult ADHD symptoms include Catapres, Tenex, and various beta blockers, including Attenolol, Inderal, Nadolol, and Metaprolol. Catapres and Tenex are sometimes prescribed to eliminate tics, impulsivity, and aggression.

These drugs require closer medical monitoring. Blood tests and sometimes an EKG may also be required.

Other Medications for Adult ADHD

A few other medications have been used to treat adult ADHD.

- Desyrel (trazodone) is a mild antidepressant that may be prescribed for those who have trouble falling asleep.
- Buspar, a serotonin stabilizer, is sometimes prescribed to control anxiety in adults with ADHD.
- Some adult women with ADHD are prescribed estrogen replacement therapy to alleviate depression and improve memory and attention span. Studies show that falling estrogen levels can exacerbate adult ADHD symptoms of depression, anxiety, and inattention. However, each woman should review the risks and benefits with her gynecologist since estrogen affects many systems in the body.

- Nicotinic analogues, or medications that act on some of the same brain receptors as nicotine, may also provide some relief. Although most research on ADHD has revolved around regulating the balance of neurotransmitters, some believe poor regulation of the nicotinic receptors may also be involved. Adults with ADHD are more likely to smoke cigarettes, and research showed improved symptoms in ADHD adults who wore the transdermal nicotine patch. More studies are needed to isolate which properties in the patch were responsible for symptom relief.

Choosing and Monitoring Your Medication

It's important to find medication(s) that not only alleviates your symptoms but facilitates your physical, emotional, and mental health. Although stimulants have long been considered first-line medications for adult ADHD, before agreeing to take a medication it's important to educate yourself on the positive and negative effects of the drug so you can make an informed decision. It's also very important to read the fine print concerning your medication, including its estimated half-life and peak time, how many doses you need to take, whether the medication is short-acting or long-acting, and whether the medication is available in extended release forms so you can take it once and forget about it. If you're suffering from coexisting conditions that complicate your adult ADHD, it's also important to take medication that controls those symptoms as well.

The Importance of Monitoring Your Meds

While monitoring the effectiveness of your medication will require some effort on your part, the results are well worth it. By keeping track of how well the drug works over time, you and your doctor can make the necessary adjustments in medications and dosages to keep you functioning at your best.

In 2007, the FDA required that all makers of ADHD medications develop patient medication guides containing information about the risks associated with the medications, including possible cardiovascular or psychiatric problems. The guides were the result of data that showed adult ADHD patients had a slightly higher risk of stroke, heart attack, and/or sudden death when taking the medications.

Those taking medication for ADHD were also slightly more at risk for medication-related psychiatric problems, such as hearing voices, having hallucinations, becoming suspicious for no reason, or becoming manic. These symptoms appeared in patients who did not have a history of psychiatric problems.

Best Ways to Take Adult ADHD Medication

To maximize the effectiveness of your medication and to minimize the side effects and risks, follow these easy guidelines for safe use.

❑ Do your homework. Find out everything you can about the ADHD medications your doctor is prescribing, including potential side effects, how often to take it, special warnings, and other medications and substances that should be avoided or used with caution such as over-the-counter cold and flu remedies containing ephedrine, over-the-counter and prescription weight-loss drugs, sleep medications, decongestants, steroids, and asthma medications containing albuterol or theophylline.

❑ Always take your medication as directed. Never take more or less than prescribed, and always take it at the exact time and in the exact way prescribed by your physician.

❑ Don't let a high-fat breakfast sabotage your medication. If you're taking certain stimulant drugs, including Adderall, Metadate, and Ritalin, a high-fat breakfast can compromise the medication's effectiveness by delaying the drug's absorption. It can take as long as two hours for the drug to work instead of the usual twenty to thirty minutes. Forgo high-fat breakfasts and stick to low-fat options like oatmeal with berries or an egg-white omelet with low-fat cheese and low-fat turkey bacon.

❏ Avoid foods and supplements high in vitamin C. Fruit juices high in ascorbic acid, vitamin C, or citric acid may interfere with the absorption of Ritalin because citric acid breaks down the medication before the body has a chance to absorb it. For this reason, your doctor may recommend you avoid fruit juices, high-vitamin cereals, and multivitamin supplements an hour before and after taking medication.

❏ Be patient. Finding the right medication and dose is a trial-and-error process. It will take some experimenting and open, honest communication with your doctor.

❏ Start small. Begin with a small dose and see how it works. The best approach may be to take the least amount necessary to get beneficial results.

❏ Keep records of how the medication is affecting your emotions, behavior, attention, sleep, appetite, weight, and other aspects of your life. Keep track of any unusual or new side effects that occur, and keep an ongoing record of how effective the medication seems to be in alleviating your symptoms.

❏ Don't stop a drug cold turkey because it is ineffective or has unpleasant side effects. You could suffer from discontinuation syndrome, and symptoms like depression, irritability, fatigue, insomnia, and headaches could last for weeks.

Remember that medication is just one side of your treatment triangle. By recording your reactions to drugs on a regular basis, it will be easier to isolate unusual emotional, mental, and physical symptoms that appear to be linked to medication. You'll also be able to identify persisting symptoms that may benefit from other types of treatment, such as cognitive or support psychotherapy, coaching, and support groups.

Positive and Negative Effects of Medication

Sometimes it can be hard to figure out what constitutes a positive reaction to a drug. Is it the medication or something else that is making you feel better? Which negative side effects are worth mentioning to your physician?

Zoning in on Positive Results

Your reaction may be immediate or gradual, but suddenly you're positive you've got a handle on your adult ADHD symptoms. You're not only thinking and acting better, but you're feeling better.

In fact, there are many signs that your medication is working. They include being better able to pay attention, feeling less distracted, being better able to recall things, getting things done on time more often, feeling less restless and jittery, tending to think before you speak instead of blurting things out, having more control over your emotions and moods, suffering fewer and less severe mood swings, displaying less erratic behavior, being more motivated, having an easier time starting and finishing projects, getting a better night's sleep, enjoying a better sex life, finding it easier to make and keep friends, and feeling less tempted to engage in reckless behavior.

One caveat to remember if your medication program appears to be working: Don't assume that just because you're feeling better, you can take less medication or, conversely, that taking more medication will make you feel even better. There's a very small difference between the right dose and too little or too much medication, so resist the temptation to experiment on your own. Include your doctor in your plans and discuss your experience with him.

Noting Negative Side Effects

Although every medication has side effects, not everyone has the same reactions to them. Some people may barely notice side effects while others may be so bothered by them that they have to take a lower dosage or stop taking the drug altogether. If you suffer from one or more of the following side effects, contact your doctor.

- Personality changes. If you're normally sunny and upbeat and you suddenly become all doom and gloom, it may be time to switch to another medication.
- Trouble falling asleep. While insomnia is a fairly common problem among adults with ADHD, if your medication makes things even worse ask your physician to adjust or reduce your dosage, prescribe ADHD medications with sedating qualities right before bedtime, or prescribe a sleep aid to help you fall and stay asleep.
- Rebound effects. The majority of adults who take stimulants experience rebound effects of moodiness, irritability, and restlessness as the level of medication in their bloodstream decreases. Ask your doctor about ways to stabilize the level of medication in your body to avoid these fluctuations.
- Appetite and weight loss. Many medications for adult ADHD cause a reduction in appetite and subsequent weight loss. Ask your doctor about timing your doses so your medication doesn't ruin your appetite for meals. If you're losing weight despite your best efforts, consider consulting with a registered dietitian or nutritionist.
- Aches, pains, and tics. In some adults, ADHD medications can trigger nausea, indigestion, and headaches. To ward off stomachaches, take medication with meals. If medication worsens symptoms of a coexisting condition like Tourette's syndrome, call your doctor.
- Rashes and skin disturbances. Many adults are allergic to the dyes and even the cellulose fillers in pills and react by

breaking out in a rash. To avoid future rashes, switch to a medication that doesn't have the offending culprit.

- Rapid heart beat or increased blood pressure. If you feel like your heart is racing, you can't catch your breath, you experience chest pains, or if your usual workout suddenly feels a lot more difficult, it may be a sign that you're taking too much medication.

If your medication isn't working, has stopped working, or your dose needs to be fine-tuned, you may feel anxious, depressed, jittery, restless, or unable to sleep; develop new symptoms you never experienced before; and experience inexplicable mood swings that seem to worsen no matter what you do.

In some cases, side effects are your body's way of announcing that you and the drug are not compatible. In others, these side effects are simply a temporary manifestation. In either case, you'll want to keep your physician abreast of them.

Side Effects Aren't a Life Sentence

If side effects are seriously interfering with your life, don't worry that you're stuck with them for life. There are many alternatives and "fixes," from changing medication and dosage to taking a drug holiday and trying again later. You may also consider consulting with other medical experts to get a fresh point of view about medications and treatments you haven't yet tried.

The good news is that side effects of adult ADHD medications tend to be mild and temporary. In many cases, negative side effects simply go away within a few weeks. Most of those that don't go away on their own can be eliminated by simply changing the dosage or dosage schedule, or by switching to a new medication.

CHAPTER 10

Exploring the Benefits of Talk Therapy

Although medications for treating adult ADHD have proven to be very successful in reducing symptoms, they can't teach new skills or improve the organizational and interpersonal challenges that usually accompany the disorder. Talk therapy takes many forms, but it always involves talking with a trained therapist. Depending on the specific type of talk therapy, you'll learn about the neurobiological natures of the disorder, stop blaming yourself for your symptoms, and develop new tools and strategies for coping with everyday symptoms of adult ADHD at home, at work, and in social settings.

Why Talk Therapy Works

Everyone needs someone to talk to, whether they are going through a major life challenge like adult ADHD or just trying to figure out how to cope with a minor setback. Adults with ADHD have myriad issues to contend with, from the symptoms of the disorder to the isolating nature of the condition. Psychotherapy gives you the coping skills you need to live with the disorder. Although very few studies of psychotherapy and adult ADHD have been conducted, several published trials indicate that up to 70 percent of adults who undergo various types of psychotherapy as well as take medication show a dramatic improvement in symptoms of anxiety and depression.

It's important to remember that adult ADHD has no ultimate cure. While neither medication nor psychotherapy can completely eliminate the symptoms of adult ADHD, psychotherapy can help you understand, manage, and minimize your symptoms so they are less likely to negatively impact your life.

Types of Psychotherapy

Just as there are many different regimens for weight loss, there are many different types of therapy. Some focus on helping you come to a better understanding of why you think, act, and feel differently than "normal" people. Others help you adjust your behavior, emotions, and thinking so they don't sabotage your personal relationships, your ability to get or keep a job, or your unique talent to create startling new concepts.

In general, psycho-education and talk therapy can help you deal with feelings of low self-esteem, inadequacy, anxiety, depression, and underachievement. Behavioral and skills-training therapy are useful in helping developing new ways to deal with specific issues, rebuild organizational and planning skills, and learn time management and effective communication skills.

Although most therapists emphasize one approach over another, the best therapists are able to combine elements of talk, behavioral, and skills therapy and use them interchangeably depending on the specific situation and circumstances.

Learning Through Psychoeducation

If you've never been in therapy before and have just been diagnosed with adult ADHD, psychoeducation therapy is often a good place to start. In this type of therapy, your counselor acts more like an instructor than a therapist to teach you about the disorder.

You'll learn that all those symptoms you always thought to be "your fault," or caused by innate laziness, stupidity, lack of motivation, or disinterest, are actually the result of a neurobiological imbalance of neurotransmitters that control attention and impulse. You'll also learn why it's harder for you than others to pay attention, focus, remember things, get things done on time, start things, prioritize, and know when to shift gears.

Learning and understanding the biological roots of adult ADHD can also help you begin to banish years of guilt and blame and open the floodgates for seeking the help you need to overcome symptoms.

Skills-Training Therapy

Adults with ADHD often feel as though their lives are in disarray. Skills-training helps adults with ADHD develop the executive skills they need to function more effectively at work and at home.

⌂. Essential

Disorganization is one of the biggest problems facing adults with ADHD. If your home is so cluttered and disorganized you routinely get late bill notices, or if you start projects but can't complete them because you misplace important documents, a professional organizer can provide the hands-on help you need to get your life and work in order.

Skills-training helps replace inefficient habits with more effective ones. It teaches ADHD adults how to enhance their organizational skills through the use of time management skills, audio and visual cues, electronic organizers, date books, calendars, lists, and methods of structuring tasks.

Types of Group Counseling

In addition to individual types of counseling, adults with ADHD often find family, group, or couples counseling very helpful as well. In group counseling, people with a common issue meet together with a therapist. Interacting with others and hearing their problems can help reduce your feelings of isolation and give you the motivation needed to change troublesome ways of thinking, feeling, and acting.

In couples therapy, also called marriage therapy, couples focus on relationship issues and problems caused by adult ADHD. The counselor may act as a psychoeducator as well as a mediator to help non-ADHD partners understand the nature of the disorder so they don't mistake symptoms for laziness, inconsiderateness, or lack of interest. In addition, therapists can help couples find acceptable compromises where there are conflicts.

Couples therapy may also address problems with intimacy and sexual dysfunction as they relate to the various symptoms of adult ADHD or medications used to treat the condition.

In family therapy, the entire family works with a counselor to fully understand the nature of adult ADHD. Family members who don't have ADHD will learn why their ADHD relatives think, act, and feel the way they do. Therapy can be instrumental in overcoming misunderstandings, changing the family's patterns of blame, and helping the family make adjustments.

Fact

Because adults with ADHD often feel awkward in social settings and have a tendency to interrupt or butt into conversations, group therapy can be a safe place to develop and practice appropriate social skills and get moral support and feedback from fellow ADHD adults.

In parenting therapy, you and your spouse learn to identify ways that adult ADHD affects your ability to be a consistent and effective parent. You also work on ways to overcome challenges presented by the disorder, such as discipline, planning, and organizing. This type of training is especially important if both you and your spouse have adult ADHD and/or if you also have children with the syndrome.

In therapy that focuses on friendships and relationships, you learn how to manage ADHD symptoms that may be affecting your ability to develop and maintain meaningful relationships, act appropriately during casual dating, feel comfortable in social settings, and work well with people on the job.

Learning to Change Your Behavior

In cognitive behavioral therapy (CBT), you and your therapist focus on the present. CBT helps you alter challenging behavior patterns, such as procrastination, smoking, and drinking, and can also be used to address conditions like depression and anxiety.

Adjuncts to Therapy

In addition to psychotherapy, adult ADHD coaches can help patients identify their goals and stay on track. Although coaches are not usually trained counselors, they can be highly effective in helping adults develop hands-on tools for managing day-to-day organizational challenges.

Adult ADHD support groups can also be therapeutic. They give people a place to share their stories, challenges, resources and coping strategies, and find solutions and support for overcoming mutual struggles.

The Benefits of Talk Therapy

As one of the oldest types of therapy, talk therapy is exactly what the name implies: It's an extended conversation between you and your therapist, with the goal of helping you better understand why you think, act, and behave the way you do.

Talk therapy can take many different forms. Throughout insight therapy, you examine your motives and your past behavior for "ah-ha" moments. During support therapy, you and your therapist look for ways to bolster your self-esteem and rein in negative thinking. During group therapy, you address adult ADHD problems as they affect your ability to have healthy interpersonal relationships with your family, your spouse or significant other, your children, and your friends.

Insight or Psychodynamic Therapy

The underlying premise of insight therapy is that our actions are the result of many conscious and unconscious factors, some of which likely stem from childhood experiences your conscious mind may have completely forgotten about, but you still react to on an emotional level. The goal of insight therapy is to uncover the motivating factors behind what you do, and find ways to adjust them for better results.

Alert

Talk therapy isn't always a walk in the park. Oftentimes, delving into your past to try to make sense of your present behavior can uncover thoughts, emotions, and memories you've suppressed for years because they were too painful to remember. A trained therapist can help you deal with painful recollections and find ways to learn and grow from them.

For instance, maybe you routinely put off paying bills until the very last minute—or until your providers turn off the water, electricity, and gas, and you're forced to make a payment.

Why you do this is another story. Are you putting it off because you can't find the bills, hate the drudgery of putting the bill in the mailbox, or because not paying the bills creates a sense of excitement and drama?

You may have deeper or hidden motives for not paying the bills on time. Maybe you unconsciously resent your wife for making you pay the bills and think she should do it instead of you. Or maybe paying the bills makes you feel anxious and insecure because they remind you that you're not earning as much money as you know you could be making.

Fortunately, an insight therapist is trained to listen closely and carefully to your real and fabricated problems and excuses and help you untangle them so you can come up with a solution to the problem before it destroys your home and marital life.

It could be as easy as making sure all the bills are in one place so you can find and pay them promptly, or putting visual cues on your computer or refrigerator to remind you that bills are due. If you're avoiding the bills to create excitement, your therapy can help you find more productive ways to create drama in your life that won't create household chaos.

On the other hand, if you're not paying the bills because you resent your wife for making you pay them, your therapist may recommend you both see a couples counselor so you can air your differences and get to the root of the problem.

Your therapist might not always be able to help you correct or eliminate the problem at hand, but he will probably be able to help you arrive at a compromise that you and your loved ones can tolerate and live with.

Focus on Supportive Therapy

If an insight therapist serves as a detective to help you uncover and understand unconscious motives, a support therapist acts more like your personal cheerleader.

After years of living with the disappointment, rejection, and failure of ADHD, you may feel like you need someone to help you pick yourself up and dust yourself off.

Alert

Support therapy requires time and patience. You didn't become negative overnight, and you're not going to emerge from your therapist's office with the positive, radiant glow of Deepak Chopra until you've learned how to stop your negative self-thoughts in their tracks and replace them with self-affirming thoughts and feelings.

Many ADHD adults are also mired in negative, doom-and-gloom thinking, primarily because they've spent a large part of their lives internalizing the reams of criticism hurled their way because of their ADHD symptoms.

If you're one of them, a support therapist can help you replace your negative thoughts, self-criticism, and low self-esteem with strategies that lead to more positive thinking. Here are some tried-and-true strategies support therapists use to help patients derail negative thoughts and a poor self-image.

- Catch yourself in the act: The minute you start thinking something negative about yourself, imagine it's a beast dragging you down to the pits. Becoming more aware of your negative thoughts can help you gain the upper hand on them.

- Stop playing that broken record in your head: When you repeatedly tell yourself "basic truths" you believe are true about yourself, such as, "I'm too dumb to be employed" or "I always screw things up with women," the limiting self-talk can make you give up before you even try. Your therapist can help you practice saying affirmative things to yourself that are probably a lot truer than those old, negative songs that have been on auto play for years now.

- Get some perspective: Another problem with ADHD adults is their tendency to magnify their own shortcomings. Maybe you always think you're to blame, no matter what the situation, or you emphasize the negative and eliminate the positive when it comes to your past and present accomplishments. As an objective party, your therapist can give you the reality check you need to readjust your attitudes about yourself.

- Learn to reframe: Just like a beautiful picture frame can enhance rather than obscure the beauty of a painting, putting a positive spin on things can turn a mistake into an opportunity for improvement. So you forgot to pick up the dry cleaning? Instead of telling yourself you're so stupid you can't remember simple errands, state the obvious in a nonjudgmental way: "I forgot to pick up the laundry." Then ask yourself what you can do to remember to pick it up tomorrow.

- Get rid of the absolutes: If you're constantly beating yourself up for "always" being late, or "never" remembering important dates, focus on the many things in life you do right. Replaying that endless (inaccurate) record in your head that says you do "everything" wrong is the sort of negative reinforcement you need to banish from your life.

- Be nice to yourself: As an ADHD adult, you've already had your share of self-criticism and rejection. It's time to treat yourself right. Work with your therapist to find ways to nurture your soul, whether it's listening to inspiring music, reading empowering books, taking a restorative walk through nature, or getting a relaxing massage.

Improving your self-image takes time and patience, but once you get the ball rolling, your positive self-talk is likely to become a self-fulfilling prophecy. As you gain self-confidence and self-respect, you'll make changes to improve the quality of your life, feel better about yourself in return, and success will beget success.

Couples and Relationship Therapy

As most of you already know, being married or involved in an intimate relationship is enough of a challenge without the added strain of adult ADHD symptoms. In couples counseling, a therapist works with you and your spouse or significant other to address problems caused by the myriad symptoms of adult ADHD.

In the typical adult ADHD marriage, the non-ADHD spouse attempts to overcompensate for the adult ADHD spouse by doing all the things her spouse forgets or neglects to do, whether it's raising the kids, making dinner, taking out the garbage, or all three.

In time, the non-ADHD spouse may start to feel more like a parent than a loving partner, and it's not unusual for resentment and frustrations to build, tempers to flare, sexual passions to wither, and the marriage to land on the rocks.

Without a therapist's intervention, being married to someone with adult ADHD can feel like living inside a three-ring minus the ringmaster. Chronic clutter, disorganization, disrepair, financial problems, unpaid bills, un- or under-employment, health issues, traffic accidents, drug and alcohol abuse, license suspensions, absentee parenting and discipline skills, children who are AWOL from school, separation, divorce, and child custody fights are just some of the issues a couple dealing with ADHD must handle.

Because most marital problems in adult ADHD marriages stem from the ADHD partner's inherent inabilities and impairments rather than laziness, lack of motivation, disinterest, or lack of desire, couples therapy usually begins by educating the non-ADHD spouse about the neurobiological roots of the disorder.

Fact

The biggest culprit of some couples' sexual problems is waning levels of ADHD medication. If your ADHD spouse is usually in the mood at night, know that waning levels of ADHD medication in his bloodstream may be the culprit behind his unfiltered thoughts and impulsive acts that throw a bucket of cold water on your libido.

Although symptoms displayed by ADHD spouses are as widely varied as the spouses who present them, many couples dealing with ADHD deal with similar problems. Just a few of them include:

❑ Spouses lost in space: Because a husband with ADHD may be highly imaginative and restless, he may find it hard to focus on or remember the necessary steps involved in successful lovemaking. G-spot? What's that? With his natural tendency toward restlessness and impulsiveness, an ADHD husband could be a speed demon in bed who's there one minute and gone the next, too hyperactive to enjoy fore-play and cuddling, and prone to ruining the moment with un-romantic comments like, "Wow, you're getting chunky!"

❏ Spouses who are hypersensitive to touch: Many adults with ADHD are annoyed or irritated by being touched in the wrong way, at the wrong time, or over too long a period of time. Make sure you communicate your likes and dislikes to each other, and remember—practice makes perfect.

❏ Spouses who routinely tune you out and forget: Glazing over when a spouse is ranting and raving about a bad day at work, or routinely forgetting important days in her life like her birthday, your anniversary, etc., can leave a non-ADHD spouse wonder why she got married in the first place if she always feels so alone anyhow. A therapist can remind the non-ADHD spouse that her husband's inattention and for-getfulness is a symptom of the disorder rather than an indi-cation he no longer cares. The therapist can also work with the husband to develop remembering cues and strategies.

❏ Spouses who fly off the handle at the slightest thing: Living with an ADHD spouse with a short temper can leave a non-ADHD spouse feel like she's tiptoeing through a mine field or living with a ticking time bomb. Because a non-ADHD spouse never knows what's going to set off her ADHD spouse next, she may avoid conversation and emotionally with-draw. One solution is for the non-ADHD spouse to simply leave the room when her spouse's temper flares. Another is for the ADHD spouse to find techniques to control his rage.

Studies show that marriages in which one or more partners have ADHD are at greater risk for domestic abuse, separation, and divorce than marriages where spouses don't have the disorder. For more infor-mation on dealing with adult ADHD in marriage, see Chapter 18.

Family Therapy

Living with a spouse with adult ADHD can translate into household chaos, especially if the non-ADHD spouse is working fulltime while still handling the brunt of the parenting, homework, and bookkeeping. If he's also saddled with household chores his ADHD spouse routinely neglects or forgets to do, it won't take long for tempers to flare and trouble to erupt.

Therapists can help couples and families organize the household so the ADHD spouse functions more effectively on a daily basis. They can also remove some burdens from the non-ADHD spouse so he feels more like a husband and less like a mother.

⌐ Essential

Establishing a family calendar where everyone puts crucial dates, doctor appointments, social engagements, social events, birthdays, and anniversaries in one central location can help relieve the non-ADHD spouse from having to serve as the family "memory bank." Remembering every detail of the family's comings and goings is a chore that can breed exhaustion, frustration, and resentment.

Visual and auditory cues, such as Post-It notes, lists, and alarms, can also help keep things on track. Creating orderly routines may also help rein in chaos. While non-ADHD people find it easy to establish and automatically follow routines, for many adults with ADHD there is no such thing as an automatic routine.

Your therapist can help you and your ADHD spouse create simple routines that will help keep household clutter and chaos in check. For instance, an ADHD husband might establish the routine of dumping the contents of his pockets in a basket by the door before he enters the house so his wallet, glasses, keys, etc., don't get scattered all over the house.

Building Better Friendships

Making and keeping friends can be very difficult for adults with ADHD. Because of their long history of misunderstanding others, confusing communication cues, and being unable to read and translate nonverbal cues, they are likely to withdraw from social interaction and feel more comfortable alone than with others.

In fact, many adults with ADHD never get the chance to establish meaningful relationships because their behavior often drives potential friends and lovers away.

 Fact

> Research shows that ADHD adults get along best with friends who are low-maintenance, don't expect or need regular contact, and who are nonjudgmental. If you have an ADHD friend who feels like she's "drifted" away, make sure you're not overestimating her ability to maintain regular contact.

Because of their forgetfulness, ADHD adults may also forget about friends' needs, and fail to do the many little things required to keep a friendship going and growing. Adults with ADHD might not call their friends on the phone, send a friendly e-mail to check on them, remember their birthdays, congratulate them on promotions, or console them in the face of job loss or the death of a loved one.

Sorry, No Time for You

Some ADHD adults, especially hyperactive adults, manifest their symptoms by jumping into conversations and situations where they're not invited, constantly interrupting others, or behaving in a hostile, arrogant or aggressive fashion—all behaviors that tend to alienate people.

Your therapist and you can work together on strategies that will help you check your impulses before making grandiose promises you can't keep. She can encourage you to learn how to say "no" when someone's expectations are impossible for you to meet, and to compensate for your inherent tendency toward aloofness and solitude by making a conscious attempt to be more interested and engaged in the lives of others.

Parenting Therapy

In addition to wreaking havoc on marriage and friendships, adult ADHD traits such as intolerance for boredom and routine and a need for constant excitement, stimulation, and action, can interfere with the ability to be a responsive and responsible parent.

Studies show that many adults with ADHD have erratic parenting styles. They tend to be inconsistent in terms of establishing discipline, setting goals, and maintaining realistic expectations, a fact that often results in household confusion and chaos.

 Alert

Many adults with ADHD are too distracted, disorganized, and forgetful to perform the most routine household chores and tasks, such as helping a child with homework, preparing dinner, or taking a child to an after-school activity. Over time, the household unravels into unending chaos, clutter, and disarray that disrupt the lives of everyone in the family.

Parents with ADHD may also be too restless, impatient, or hyperactive to bond with children in time-honored ways, such as reading a storybook to a child at bedtime, playing simple board games with children in the evening, or watching a child's favorite TV show with him.

Strategies for Improving Parenting Skills

Parenting therapists can help you identify and begin to correct parenting behavior that may be adversely affecting your child, as well as your relationship with your child, by helping you find new parenting modes that tap into your strengths (creativity, spontaneity) and minimize your shortcomings (low threshold for boredom, impatience, desire for constant stimulation and excitement).

Spending more time doing creative things with your children that you actually enjoy, such as building things, cooking, or planning a garden, can improve the quality of the time you spend with them.

If a child wants to do an activity that you find dull or boring, you can either find a new and more exciting way to approach the game or project, or agree to the request but limit the time period.

The Role of Coaches and Support Groups

Although coaching, like therapy, revolves around talking, unlike therapy, coaching is aimed at helping adults develop practical, concrete tools for dealing with the challenges of the disorder. Instead of delving into the past for hidden reasons or motivations behind why you may behave the way you do, a coach focuses on the present.

If you have trouble starting projects, instead of exploring and analyzing the many reasons why you may avoid doing a specific job, a coach focuses on helping you develop specific strategies to eliminate procrastination, such as breaking a large task down into small bites and using visual cues and reminders to stay on track.

Gaining Insight Through Support Groups

Many ADHD adults avoid social situations and, as a result, become isolated and out of touch. Support groups can provide ADHD adults with a safe place to develop and practice social skills in a supportive, nonjudgmental, and caring environment.

By sharing their stories and learning that others share the same difficulties, ADHD adults can help overcome the feelings of isolation that often make them feel like social outcasts and build the supportive relationships they need to carry them through challenging times.

You'll get the best support from your group if you know the ground rules going in and understand that being part of a support group entails listening as well as talking. It's also very important to understand the structure of your support group and how it functions. Some groups combine casual socializing with collective sharing during the meeting, while others set aside opportunities to socialize and mingle before and/or after the official meeting.

Essential

Remember that an adult ADHD support group isn't an excuse to "let it all hang out," but an opportunity to share mutual problems and build on your social skills in a supportive setting. Make sure your impulsivity doesn't cause you to chatter away without thinking and self-censoring, or that your hyperactivity doesn't leave you jumping into conversations before you're invited.

For best results, test the waters when you first join a support group before taking the plunge. Sit quietly and observe for the first few meetings before actively participating. Sharing too much about yourself may make you feel uncomfortable later, while sharing too little may make you seem indifferent or bored to others in the group.

Take your cues from others to find the right balance between talking and listening, but a good rule of thumb is to listen more than you talk and contribute only when you have something concrete and appropriate to say.

By joining a support group, you've made an unwritten agreement to listen as well as talk, and to view the support group as a tool for helping yourself as well as others gain insight and find solutions to adult ADHD-related challenges and problems.

CHAPTER 11

Weighing the Role of Behavioral Modification

C hanging your adult ADHD behavior is probably your biggest priority, and behavioral modification is another tool that can help you attain that goal. Developed during the 1950s by researchers looking for an alternative to talk therapy, behavioral modification focuses on the here-and-now and employs a variety of techniques that help you reinforce positive behavior and reduce undesirable behavior. Cognitive behavioral therapy and interpersonal therapy are other types of behavioral modification used to treat adult ADHD. Studies show behavioral modification is most effective when combined with medication and psychotherapy.

Three Types of Behavioral Modification

The goal of behavioral modification is to help you develop new tools and strategies for developing better behavioral patterns, and to help you become more adept at learning from the results of your actions. In fact, behavioral therapists believe that other therapies are effective because they unknowingly benefit from behavioral principles.

Of course, talk is still required during behavior modification therapy. But in behavioral modification, communication of information is not the essence of the approach. In fact, the behavioral therapy approach suggests that the cognitive and psychic aspects of therapy are over-valued.

Traditional Behavioral Modification

While traditional behavioral modification is widely used in treating children with ADHD, its use in adults has become more limited since the advent of cognitive-behavioral therapy and interpersonal therapy. Today, parents and teachers use traditional behavioral therapy for encouraging good study habits and discouraging misbehavior in children and students. Behavioral modification is most often used in a highly structured situation or environment in which rewards are used to reinforce positive behavior and consequences are used to discourage negative behavior.

Cognitive Behavioral Therapy

Cognitive behavioral therapy (CBT) is a type of psychotherapy that helps you change the way you think, feel, or act so you can improve your mood, reduce stress, or achieve other important health and life goals.

Your goals can be as specific as reducing feelings of awkwardness in a particular social setting, or as general as figuring out why your life feels meaningless and what you can do to change it. CBT is widely regarded as one of the most promising new forms of behavior modification for treating adult ADHD.

Interpersonal Therapy

Although interpersonal therapy (IPT) is similar to CBT in that it addresses present-day behavior, unlike CBT it looks at how problems with personal relationships can cause you to become depressed or make your existing depression even worse. Because IPT helps you shift the blame of depression from yourself to your disorder and the interpersonal problem, it is also helpful in alleviating feelings of blame or guilt.

Unlike other types of behavioral modification, which may last for several months, IPT is limited to between twelve and sixteen sessions. While no studies have examined the effectiveness of IPT on adults with ADHD, many therapists and patients consider it a highly useful adjunct to medication because the disorder usually causes interpersonal problems in marriages and relationships.

Adult ADHD and Behavioral Modification

Behavior is a highly complicated process. Put simply, it involves two distinct steps: feed forward and feedback. During the feed-forward stage, you think about what you want to do, then do it. For instance, you decide you're hungry, so you make a sandwich and eat it to satisfy your hunger. During the feedback stage, you evaluate how well your plan of action worked and make necessary adjustments or corrections. For instance, you figure out if eating a sandwich satisfied your hunger. If it didn't, you make another sandwich and eat it.

The Problem with Feedback in Adult ADHD

If you have adult ADHD, your brain's feed-forward and feedback processes may not be operating in the right way. While you probably have no trouble deciding you're hungry and that you need to make a sandwich, you may have trouble following through on your decision, evaluating whether you did the right thing, and figuring how to correct it if you didn't do the right thing.

Alert

Because many adults with ADHD never accomplish their original goals, they often repeat their mistakes and find it hard to behave correctly or correct behaviors that aren't working. Over time, behavioral modification can help you reshape your behavior by rewarding you for positive outcomes and delivering consequences for negative behavior.

For instance, a person without adult ADHD would get hungry, make a sandwich, and feel satisfied. But an adult with ADHD may encounter various distractions along the way. She may get too distracted to make a sandwich and impulsively wolf down a bag of corn chips instead, slap together a sandwich that doesn't really satisfy what she was craving, decide it's too much trouble to make a sandwich and simply ignore her hunger, or binge on one sandwich after another.

Using Behavioral Modification to Build Executive Functions

Behavioral modification can help adults with ADHD develop and manage organizational and executive skills. To compensate for their lack of executive function, many ADHD adults develop ineffective and idiosyncratic habits in an effort to cope with everyday tasks. Behavioral modification can help them restructure and reorder their work and home environments to increase efficiency and reduce chaos and clutter.

Focus on Traditional Behavioral Modification

Behavioral modification is based on a number of different theories and research studies. It was influenced by the classical conditioning principles set forth by Russian physiologist Ivan Pavlov, theories set forth by American B. F. Skinner, and the work of psychiatrist Joseph Wolpe.

Pavlov was most famous for training dogs to salivate at the sound of a bell—a case of rewarding and shaping behavior that usually cannot be deliberately controlled. Pavlov demonstrated how such learned responses can be suppressed. This has implications for treating emotional reactions.

Skinner was a pioneer in the field of operant conditioning, which believes that behavior generally understood as conscious and intentional is modified by changing the response it elicits. Wolpe was famous for his pioneering efforts in the areas of desensitization and assertiveness training. By the 1970s, behavior therapy was widely used in treating a variety of mental conditions, including depression, anxiety, phobias, and ADHD.

While many therapists today who treat adult ADHD have switched to CBT or IPT therapy, traditional behavioral modification remains popular for treating children with ADHD and is also very effective in institutional settings such as prisons, which are already highly structured and where rewards and punishments can take the form of basic life needs like meals and exercise.

Cognitive Behavioral Therapy

CBT was developed by psychologist Aaron Beck and others in the 1960s and is based on the idea that ineffective and self-defeating behavior is caused by "automatic thoughts," or what Beck defined as inappropriate and irrational thinking patterns. When you react to automatic thoughts, you're responding to your own imagined or distorted version of reality instead of to what's actually happening or being said.

In CBT, you learn how to change automatic thoughts that result in distorted views by examining what you consider real and valid. Your therapist uses a process called cognitive restructuring to help you cross-examine these thoughts.

 Fact

Because CBT is employed for so many different disorders, including adult ADHD, and is usually used in conjunction with medications and other treatment interventions, it has been difficult to measure its overall success rate. However, several studies have indicated that CBT is one of the most effective behavior modification treatments for adult ADHD, especially when combined with pharmacotherapy.

Some adults with ADHD have so many "automatic beliefs" that their core beliefs are flawed and negatively impact their ability to function effectively. In cases like these, therapists must work from the ground up to help patients establish new ways of thinking and behaving, a process that can take years to kick in.

How CBT Works

If you have adult ADHD, you may be convinced you have a constellation of traits that make you unlovable, unpleasant, difficult to live with, impossible to work with, and hard to get along with. You may withdraw from society because you believe it's easier to remain alone than struggle to get along with others.

CBT therapists generally work on one behavioral trait at a time. Let's say you're a single man with adult ADHD who assumes women don't want to be around you because you're overly blunt and sloppy—two traits that are very common among adult men with ADHD.

Your therapist would put your basic assumption to the test by asking you to name some women friends and family members who enjoy being around you and who have not abandoned you because you speak your mind and sometimes forget to comb your hair or change your shirt.

Fact

Other behavioral techniques used in CBT may include conditioning, or using positive and/or negative reinforcement to encourage a desired behavior, and systematic desensitization, or gradually exposing you to situations that create anxiety in order to reduce or quiet your fear response.

By showing you that there are women in your life who like you and who haven't deserted you, your therapist can expose your irrational assumption that "no woman wants to be around me because I'm blunt and sloppy." This gives you a new model of thought so you can change your previous thought pattern to one that sounds something like this: "I'm a likable and lovable guy who many women love to be around, despite the fact that I can be overly blunt and am sometimes sloppy. Therefore, though not all women will respond to me, I expect to be able to find women to go out with. Things are not as bad as I thought."

Alert

CBT is a team effort between you and your therapist, so it's essential you feel comfortable with your therapist and regard her as someone you can trust. Before committing to several sessions, schedule a consultation visit with your prospective therapist to ensure you're compatible and that she has the credentials and experience you're looking for.

While CBT sessions are usually held in a therapist's office or clinic, it's also possible to arrange for group sessions. Your therapist should be licensed in your state for independent practice; have specialty training in CBT; and be a psychologist with a PhD, PsyD, or EdD, a clinical social worker with an MSW, DSW, or LSW degree, or a psychiatrist with an MD. Your best bet is a licensed PhD-level psychologist.

CBT Techniques

Your therapist is likely to use a variety of different techniques during the course of therapy to help you transform flawed assumptions into valid ones. Here are some popular strategies used by CBT therapists.

- Validity testing. Your therapist will ask you to prove your mistaken thought or belief about yourself. If you can't offer concrete evidence to show your belief is correct or accurate, he exposes your "fact" as a falsehood you've been repeating to yourself.

- Cognitive rehearsal. Your therapist asks you to describe a difficult situation in the past that you responded to in an inappropriate or ineffective way. Then, using suggestions provided by your counselor, you role play the right response until it becomes habit. The next time the problem arises in your life, you can use your rehearsed behavior to cope with it more effectively.
- Guided discovery. Just as geologists use topographic maps to find earthquake faults, your therapist asks you a series of questions designed to help you uncover a cognition distortion or falsehood you've been assuming about yourself or your life.
- Journal writing. Your therapist will ask you to write down a detailed account of situations that come up in everyday life, along with how you were thinking, feeling, and behaving at the time. By reviewing your journal, you and your therapist can find patterns of distorted thinking that may be leading to your faulty thoughts and behavior.
- Reinforcing through homework. To help you continue uncovering the falsehoods you've been telling yourself in your daily life and to reinforce concepts you've learned in therapy, your therapist may give you a variety of simple homework assignments. They may range from taking notes during therapy and transcribing them into your journal after the session to reading books and articles that shed additional light on CBT or the specific issues you're dealing with. Homework may also involve practicing a new way of dealing with a problem and recording the results for discussion during the next therapy session.
- Modeling your therapist. Your therapist will role play appropriate responses to problematic situations so you can copy her response in the event the situation arises.
- Systematic reinforcement and punishment. To reduce negative behavior patterns, your therapy may deliberately with-

hold reinforcement using a method called extinction. For example, if you have a habit of interrupting conversations with her, she may ignore what you're saying every time you butt in, pretend she didn't hear you, or simply leave the room.

- Aversive conditioning. This technique borrows principles of basic conditioning to diminish the appeal of a behavior that's difficult for you to change because it's ingrained or very rewarding. During aversive conditioning, you'll be exposed to unpleasant stimulus while you're thinking about the negative behavior in question or actively engaged in that behavior. Eventually you'll come to associate the unpleasant stimulus with the activity itself and stop doing it. Aversive conditioning has been tried to help alcoholics stop drinking and to help obese people avoid some of their favorite snacks. For instance, nausea-inducing medication is administered with alcohol so a person with an alcohol problem develops an aversion to the taste and smell of alcohol. In time, the person associates alcohol with unpleasant feelings of nausea.

- Counterconditioning. This technique weakens a negative behavior by strengthening an opposite response by teaching you techniques that directly reduce panic and fear and replace them with feelings of calm and tranquility. This method is often used to treat phobias and has been very successful in programs for fearful flyers.

Interpersonal Therapy

Interpersonal therapy is one of the newest types of behavior modification being used to treat adult ADHD and is not yet widely available. Instead of learning to correct negative thoughts and behaviors, IPT focuses on helping you understand why and how your personal relationships are making you depressed. It also alleviates feelings of guilt and blame by encouraging you to shift the blame and guilt onto the disorder itself as well as the specific interpersonal situation.

Unlike other types of behavioral conditioning that may continue for months or years, IPT is a short-term therapy limited to between twelve and sixteen weeks; although new research shows that ongoing "maintenance therapy" following short-term IPT may prevent future episodes of depression, particularly in women.

However, as with other types of behavioral modification, IPT requires a commitment on the part of the patient to practice skills taught in IPT therapy. Those who don't practice are not likely to experience significant or permanent relief from symptoms and may suffer relapses.

Why IPT Is Helpful to Adults with ADHD

Interpersonal therapy is typically used in situations involving grief or loss, changing roles, and interpersonal problems with others. These are all common problem areas for adults with ADHD. Many ADHD adults suffer grief over being disabled, losing a job, or driving people away and losing friends and spouses. Because of their ADHD symptoms, they tend to change jobs more often, get fired more often, have a higher rate of divorce, and be involved in more traffic accidents and injuries, which all involve changing roles.

Fact

Because many adults with ADHD have volatile symptoms like short tempers, impatience, hyperactivity, and recklessness, they have significant trouble establishing and maintaining close relationships, tend to be socially withdrawn and isolated, and may lack social and communication skills.

In addition, interpersonal arguments and problems are the rule rather than the exception with many ADHD adults because they have difficulty getting along with everyone from casual acquaintances to spouses, family members, and close friends.

The Role of Body Awareness Training

Awareness training is any type of activity that increases your awareness of yourself in your environment. Popular types of body awareness training include meditation, martial arts, tai chi, and some types of yoga.

While body awareness therapy is a complementary or alternative therapy, many adults with ADHD find that incorporating it into their daily life helps improve their ability to pay attention and relieves stress, tension, and anxiety.

The Benefits of Walking Meditation

While there are many different types of meditation, one of the easiest for adults with ADHD to master is walking meditation. Unlike other types of meditation that require that you hold a pose—which can be difficult or impossible for hyperactive ADHD adults—walking meditation uses the natural rhythm and hypnotic pace of walking to help you relax, unwind, clear your mind, slow racing thoughts, and release negative thoughts and emotions.

While you can engage in walking meditation practically anywhere, many adults with ADHD find it especially effective when done in nature. If you live near a park or river, strolling amidst inspiring scenery can enhance the restorative effects of walking meditation and increase your overall feelings of well being. Exercise also releases endorphins, or "feel-good" hormones that temporarily elevate mood and reduce anxiety and stress.

Using Yoga and Tai Chi to Achieve Serenity

Yoga and tai chi can also help you release negative emotions by encouraging deep, steady breathing. You center your mind and focus on the present by repeating a mantra, and you enhance body awareness by slowing down and respecting your own internal rhythms. While some forms of yoga require holding a pose for long periods of time, active yoga can help you release negative emotions through action and movement. Because walking meditation, yoga, and tai chi all focus on helping you develop more awareness of your body, they keep your focus in the present and help you learn to pay attention to your feelings, thoughts, and behavior.

While body awareness training alone can't treat the symptoms of adult ADHD, because these techniques encourage you to slow racing thoughts and explore your behavior, they may complement other types of therapy in helping you replace negative thoughts and actions with positive ones.

CHAPTER 12

Healing Through Neurofeedback

Adults with ADHD have lower than normal activity in brain waves that are associated with attention and focus. During neurofeedback training, you play computer games while watching the monitor. As you improve your score in the games, you move your brain waves in a desired direction. As you repeatedly alter your brain waves to achieve a desired balance, your brain learns how to create conditions that support the re-balancing. By changing your brain function, your brain learns to compensate for adult ADHD.

Overview of Treatment

Although neurofeedback has its roots in the 1960s, it remains very controversial and still isn't universally accepted by the medical community. Critics argue there's much less scientific evidence backing neurofeedback than stimulant medication, and that it should be viewed as an experimental or alternative therapy because it offers few lasting benefits and is very expensive and time-consuming.

Proponents claim that while there are no perfectly designed studies, there is sufficient convincing research to prove that neurofeedback benefits ADHD adults, including studies that show it's even more effective than medication. Learning a little more about neurofeedback can, at the very least, assist you in making an educated decision as to whether you should incorporate it into your treatment program.

Research has already proven that a number of neurological disorders, such as epilepsy, can be characterized by distinctive EEG patterns, and that neurofeedback may help clients change those patterns.

Fact

Neurofeedback, which is also known as EEG biofeedback, is an approach for treating adult ADHD. Individuals receive real-time feedback on their brainwave activity using computer programs and learn how to alter their typical EEG pattern to one that is consistent with a more focused and attentive state.

According to neurofeedback proponents, when ADHD adults undergo the procedure they are better able to pay attention, focus, and concentrate.

Inside a Neurofeedback Session

The relaxing, noninvasive process lasts anywhere from thirty to forty-five minutes and is typically performed one to three times a week for between six and eight months. Regardless of whether you're getting neurofeedback for anxiety, depression, or adult ADHD, the procedure is relatively consistent.

Your therapist will probably begin your treatment by administering a battery of psychological and neuropsychological tests similar or identical to those you took when you were first diagnosed with adult ADHD. After your therapist analyzes test results and inputs relevant data into a computer program, you will be hooked up to an EEG machine via nineteen electrodes attached painlessly to your scalp.

The electrodes will deliver a baseline evaluation of your brain activity to the computer, which will then compare it against a data base of "normal" brain activity for people your age. Based on the data, your therapist will choose "brain exercises" designed to help you improve brain activity in areas of your brain that function in a different way from "normal" brains.

Your "brain workout" may consist of computer games you play as a computer program gauges changes made to your brain wave patterns. You may play a game where your brain waves "fly" an airplane. As you change your brain waves, you can observe the plane changing speed, altitude, and direction.

As well as helping you correct negative thought patterns, learning how to control your brain activity through neurofeedback can be very empowering, and it can help boost your self-confidence and self-esteem. Once you know you have the tools to put the brakes on runaway negative behavior and thought patterns caused by adult ADHD, you can nip destructive behavior in the bud before it has a chance to sabotage you.

A Tour of Your Brain Waves

The brain has five major types of brain wave patterns. Although there are many different patterns in your brain at any given time, these waves can reflect your existing mood or mental state.

- Beta waves are the fastest waves in your brain, and the brain waves you experience when you're awake. Brain wave frequencies are generally above 12 hertz, which are cycles of activity per second. When you're feeling alert, attentive, excited, energized, focused, or revved up, your brain is in beta wave mode. You're also in beta wave mode when you're focusing on a project at work, reading a mystery novel, doing a crossword puzzle, or watching an adventure movie.
- SMR waves, a subgroup of beta waves, occur when you're concentrating on how to prepare for a physical challenge, such as climbing a flight of steps, taking a bike ride, working out, or taking a hike or walk.
- Alpha waves are slower than beta waves and are associated with relaxing and winding down. You'd be in alpha wave mode

if you were getting a massage or listening to relaxing music. Alpha waves have frequencies ranging from 8–12 Hz. Some ADHD adults have too many alpha waves, which get in the way of normal communication between different parts of the brain.

- Theta waves are even slower than alpha waves. This is the brain pattern you're in when you're daydreaming, visualizing, meditating, or about to fall asleep. Theta wave frequencies range from 4–8 Hz. Many ADHD adults have too many theta waves. During neurofeedback, you do brain exercises to increase your level of beta waves in brain areas bogged down by theta waves.

- Delta waves are the slowest brain waves of all and the mode you're in when you're asleep. Delta brain wave frequencies range from 0–4 Hz.

Benefits of Neurofeedback

During neurofeedback, neuroelectrical activity is detected via electrodes attached to your scalp. This activity is then amplified and processed by software programs that provide auditory, tactile, and/or visual feedback to you via a game simulation or computer monitor.

When someone without adult ADHD does something that requires a lot of focus, concentration, and attention, they activate beta waves in certain parts of the brain. But ADHD adults doing the same task activate theta waves (the daydream brain wave) instead of focused beta waves. While they may have trouble paying attention to things that bore them, these same individuals may excel at things that capture their interest, such as creating new worlds for movies (Steven Spielberg), inventing a completely new way of painting (Pablo Picasso), or developing the principles behind rocket science (Isaac Newton).

Proponents of neurofeedback believe it helps ADHD adults by teaching them how to adjust their brain waves so they more closely resemble the brain waves of "normal" people.

Fact

In essence, neurofeedback is a workout for your brain. It helps strengthen the attentive, or beta wave, muscles of your brain that you'd use to do things like concentrate on your tax return, pay attention to what your wife is saying, or focus on your project at work.

How Neurofeedback Shifts Your Brain Waves

Let's say your computer "brain training" is a Pac-Man computer game. Before starting the game, your therapist establishes "amplitude thresholds" designed to help you optimize motivation and learning.

As you play the game, a Pac-Man figure advances and sounds a tone whenever you maintain waves in the 15 to 18 Hz range above a certain amplitude threshold, while keeping waves in the 4 to 7 Hz range below a certain threshold. You're rewarded whenever you maintain 15 to 18 Hz above your predetermined threshold 70 percent of the time, while keeping the 4 to 7 Hz frequency above your predetermined threshold 20 percent of the time.

To sum up, during neurofeedback, you get a visual representation of what your brain waves are up to when you're doing any given task. The more you positively reinforce your brain waves for shifting to the correct mode—beta mode—the more you retrain them to stop going into the wrong mode—theta mode. It will become easier for you to stop daydreaming and fantasizing when you really should be focusing and paying attention.

Pros, Cons, and Controversy

Although many studies have claimed to show beneficial results of neurofeedback, critics continue to argue. One argument is that there aren't enough controlled studies proving the effectiveness of neurofeedback.

A controlled study by nature relies on rigorous protocol and uncompromising controls, and is usually very expensive to conduct.

Pros of Neurofeedback

Experts on both sides of the neurofeedback fence cite plenty of arguments in their favor. Here are a few reasons why proponents believe neurofeedback should be part of your adult ADHD treatment plan.

❏ Because neurofeedback does not use drugs and is also a noninvasive procedure, it may be used by adults who may not be able to tolerate ADHD drugs or who have a history of substance abuse.

❏ In some cases, neurofeedback may be as effective as stimulants and does not have significant side effects.

❏ Neurofeedback is ideal for ADHD adults who are leery of taking stimulant medications they fear may alter their personality, disrupt their natural talent for creativity, and turn them into a pale and boring shadow of themselves.

❏ Most ADHD adults find neurofeedback to be a fun, exciting, and interesting experience.

❏ Proponents of neurofeedback claim to have a solid track record of treating a variety of conditions, including adult ADHD. They claim neurofeedback has been a successful intervention in modifying seizures, traumatic brain injury, chronic pain, autistic behaviors, migraines, depression, anxiety, addictions, and sleep problems. In addition, it has also been used to resolve reading and math disability, and has reportedly helped famous athletes, artists, and executives achieve peak performance.

❏ Some ADHD adults enjoy long-lasting positive changes after undergoing neurofeedback, including reduced negative behavior and thinking patterns, and increased self-confidence and self-esteem.

❏ When the right criteria are used to select candidates for therapy and treatment, the majority of patients completing treatment reportedly show marked improvement in brain wave function.

Disadvantages of Neurofeedback

Those who oppose or question the validity of neurofeedback believe you should approach it with caution for the following reasons.

❏ There isn't enough conclusive scientific evidence to show it really works.

❏ Unlike most ADHD medications, neurofeedback is expensive. Because it's still considered an experimental treatment by many insurance companies, you could wind up paying a substantial sum. Sessions average anywhere from $50 to $100.

❏ Neurofeedback is very time-consuming, requiring that you commit twice a week for a total of 40 sessions. You may also need booster sessions from time to time.

❏ The benefits of neurofeedback are not long-lasting.

❏ It may take months for the effects of neurofeedback to kick in.

Best Candidates for Neurofeedback

Anyone with a primary diagnosis of ADHD who has between low-average and above-average intelligence can be treated with neurofeedback, according to proponents. If you suffer from certain comorbid conditions, however, you're advised to avoid it, at least until those conditions are dealt with. These include severe depression, bipolar disorder, mental retardation, childhood psychosis, a significant seizure disorder where medications interfere with learning, and being a part of a dysfunctional family that refuses to participate in therapy.

Short- and Long-term Benefits

Short-term benefits cited by proponents of neurofeedback include improved attention, focus, and concentration; an increase in organizational skills and the ability to complete tasks; and a reduction in impulsivity and hyperactivity.

Advocates claim that long-term benefits can be wide-reaching and affect virtually every aspect of an individual's life. The benefits can include improved behavior at home, at work, and in social settings; improved aptitude when learning and mastering new skills; higher intelligence test scores; increased self-esteem, confidence, and social poise; improved job performance; increased financial stability; higher socioeconomic status; improved health; increased mental and emotional stability; better marital relationships; a lower divorce rate; more stable relationships with friends, colleagues, peers, and bosses; and greater realization of innate potential.

Choosing a Neurofeedback Therapist

Several companies are involved in the neurofeedback industry. While most sell equipment to affiliated practitioners, some are more interested in turning a profit and will sell their equipment to virtually anyone. In the wrong hands, neurofeedback programs can be an expensive and frustrating waste of time.

For that reason, it's important to exercise care when choosing a neurofeedback therapist. The practitioner should ideally be licensed in psychology or in a field related to medicine, and her license should allow for independent practice. She should also be a state-licensed, PhD-level psychologist with training in brain anatomy and function and be certified by the Behavioral Certification Institute of America. In addition, your practitioner should stay abreast of the latest research, receive ongoing training in neurofeedback, and be knowledgeable in other treatment approaches to adult ADHD.

CHAPTER 13

Weighing the Effects of Diet

E xperts generally agree that bad eating habits do not cause adult ADHD, and even eating beneficial foods can't eliminate core problems as effectively as medication, psychotherapy, and behavioral modification therapy. However, recent studies suggest that what you eat may exacerbate or worsen your existing ADHD symptoms, even if they don't actually cause or trigger them. While the jury is still out on how specific foods impact symptoms, research suggests that nutrients responsible for brain health may help stabilize mood and alleviate depression, while reducing sugar intake may decrease hyperactivity.

Pros, Cons, and Controversy

Diet is probably the most controversial issue in terms of treating and managing adult ADHD. While many studies have been conducted to determine how certain foods affect children with ADHD, very little research has been done for adult ADHD. While most ADHD experts agree than consuming a healthy diet can give your brain the nutrients it needs to function most effectively, studies have not yet proven that consuming certain nutrients will alleviate or reduce specific adult ADHD symptoms. Two of the most controversial ADHD diets are supplementation diets in which you take vitamins, minerals, and other nutrients to compensate for deficiencies allegedly caused by the neurobiological and/or lifestyle symptoms of adult ADHD, and elimination diets in which you remove offending foods or ingredients.

Because neither diet has been sanctioned by the medical community at large, both are considered experimental.

Benefits of Dietary Intervention

Brain researchers believe that what's good for the brain is also good for adult ADHD. They claim a high-protein, low-carbohydrate diet may help improve concentration and focus, and reduce the time it takes for ADHD medications to work. They advocate a diet high in beans, cheese, eggs, meat, and nuts, with a focus on protein-rich foods in the morning and afternoon to bolster concentration and increase the longevity of ADHD drugs.

They also recommend reducing your intake of sugar and simple carbohydrates to avoid sugar highs and lows that can lead to rapid mood swings, depression, and erratic behavior as well as hyperactivity, restlessness, and insomnia. You can accomplish this by limiting your consumption of candy, honey, corn syrup, snack foods, white flour products, white rice, fruits with high sugar content, and starchy vegetables like potatoes and yams.

Advocates of dietary intervention for adult ADHD recommend eating more omega-3 fatty acids, which are found in tuna, salmon, other cold-water white fish, walnuts, Brazil nuts, olive and canola oils, and in supplement form. Taking daily nutritional supplements to counteract deficiencies caused by adult ADHD is also advised.

Disadvantages of Dietary Intervention

Some experts believe restricted and special diets have little or limited affect on adults with ADHD, and that nothing can substitute for the holy trinity of medication, behavioral therapy, and psychotherapy when it comes to managing adult ADHD. According to the NIMH, there is a lot of quackery out there when it comes to non-drug adult ADHD treatments.

The NIMH is of the opinion that restricted diets, allergy treatments, and megavitamins have not been scientifically shown to be effective in treating the majority of adults with ADHD. Other ADHD treatments that lack scientific backing, according to the NIMH, include biofeedback, medicines to correct problems in the inner ear, chiropractic adjustment, bone re-alignment, treatment for yeast infection, eye training, and special colored glasses.

Foods That "Heal" Brain Cells

Many ADHD experts contend that, since there's really no harm in eating a healthy diet, erring on the side of the dietary interventionists may encourage you to eat better in general, and perhaps even expose you to healthy foods you never considered eating before.

Feeding Your Head with Omega-3s

Existing studies have shown that adults with ADHD suffer from a neurobiological disorder involving a chemical imbalance of brain neurotransmitters. New research on the neuroplasticity of the brain suggests that people can actually grow new nerve brain cells throughout their lives and enhance existing brain cells by eating the right diet. This research also shows that most people—especially those with ADHD—lack a sufficient amount of essential fatty acids in their brains.

Sixty percent of your brain is comprised of fat, most of which is omega-3 essential acids that help regulate communication between brain cells.

Numerous studies conducted on children with ADHD showed they had a lower level of essential fatty acids than normal. Other research indicated that reduced levels of these acids resulted in learning difficulties, behavior problems, short tempers, and sleep disorders—all problems associated with ADHD.

Because your body does not make essential fatty acids, you have to consume a sufficient amount every day to nourish your brain. The best sources of omega-3 fatty acids are cold-water fish and seafood, such as salmon, herring, tuna, cod, flounder, trout, and shrimp. Other sources of essential fatty acids include nuts, soybeans, walnut oil, olive oil, and flaxseed oil.

The Importance of Amino Acids

In addition to omega-3 acids, amino acids may also help nourish your brain cells. As the building blocks of protein in your body, amino acids are the fuel that feeds your brain cells and regulates the production of brain neurotransmitters and enzymes responsible for communication between brain cells, cognition, and the transition from thought to action.

Excellent sources of amino acids are complete proteins such as meat, fish, eggs, dairy products, soy, and yogurt. If you don't eat meat, you can "make" a complete protein by combining brown rice with beans, seeds, or nuts.

The Role of B Vitamins

Research shows that B vitamins, like amino acids, also help create neurotransmitters that act as chemical messengers in the brain and nervous system. Some preliminary studies also suggest that deficiencies of certain nutrients, including vitamin B6, zinc, and phosphatidyl, are associated with ADHD-like symptoms. The corresponding theory speculates that correcting the deficiency might help curb symptoms.

⌐ Essential

Studies suggest that hyperactivity in ADHD children may be caused by low levels of serotonin in the brain. Children who were given B6 supplements showed a dramatic increase in serotonin levels, with a decrease in nervousness, irritability, depression, difficulty concentrating, and short-term memory loss.

Pyridoxal phosphate, a B6 member, is essential for the synthesis of the brain neurotransmitters serotonin, dopamine, and gamma-amino butyric acid (GABA).

Zinc and Phosphatidyl Serine (PS)

Some research also suggests a connection between adult ADHD and zinc deficiencies in children. One study found a link between zinc deficiency and children and adults who take stimulant medications like Ritalin.

In addition, clinical trials have shown that PS, a natural extract of lecithin, can improve cognition in ADHD children suffering from memory loss, mood, cognitive performance, and learning ability. However, no studies have been conducted on adults.

The Sugar Controversy

Although many adults with ADHD believe that consuming excess sugar exacerbates their symptoms and causes fluctuating mood swings, the scientific evidence remains mixed.

Studies published in the *New England Journal of Medicine* saw no correlation between excessive sugar consumption and adverse behavior. Research conducted at the University of North Carolina showed just the opposite—that the more sugar consumed by hyperactive people, the more destructive their behavior and the more restless they became. Research conducted at Yale University also suggested that over-consumption of sugar could exacerbate symptoms of inattention.

Fact

Despite the lack of evidence linking sugar to hyperactivity, there are some pretty good reasons to limit your consumption. Sugar has no food value, lots of calories, and may also dull your appetite for stabilizing foods that control mood and maintain healthy brain function.

Because the jury is still out on how sugar affects ADHD, the best barometer may be how you personally react to sugar. If excess sugar makes you feel jumpy, hyper, and restless, it may be a sign that sugar affects you in an adverse way. On the other hand, if you can eat lots of sugar without feeling hyper, you may be immune to its alleged "evil" effects.

How to Tame Your Sweet Tooth

If your ADHD symptoms are aggravated by sugar, reducing the amount you consume doesn't mean you can never look at a chocolate bar again. By making some simple substitutions and taking advantage of the new wave of sugar substitutes, you can get the upper hand on your out-of-control sweet tooth and enjoy some sugar in moderation. Here are some easy tips to try:

- ❑ Switch to sugarless gum. There are many delicious brands from which to choose, and, if nothing else, you won't subject your teeth to continual sugar-grinding.
- ❑ Instead of reaching for a chocolate bar, eat a handful of nuts. They'll satisfy your hunger even better than chocolate.
- ❑ Substitute veggie sticks and dips for sugary snacks like cookies and crackers.
- ❑ Instead of drinking fruit juice, switch to diet sodas or flavored waters. Or if you're hungry for fruit, eat the actual fruit instead.
- ❑ You can avoid fluctuations in sugar levels by pairing something sweet with protein. For instance, pair an apple or a pear with a chunk of Cheddar cheese for a healthful snack.

The Power of Protein

Studies show that adults with ADHD also have imbalances in their neurotransmitters, or the chemical messengers responsible for transmitting messages from one part of the brain to another.

Neurotransmitters are responsible for regulating your level of alertness or sleepiness. Some, like dopamine and norepinephrine, are responsible for keeping you awake, while others, like serotonin, have a calming effect that helps you fall asleep.

Research shows that protein helps regulate the neurotransmitters responsible for feeling alert. For this reason, eating meals that are high in protein can help you stay energized and focused. In addition, eating a protein-rich breakfast can prevent your ADHD medication from being absorbed too quickly, which can make you feel hyper and grumpy.

Protein Buffering

The average adult requires between 45 and 70 grams of protein a day. An ounce of cheese provides seven grams of protein, so you can see that meeting your daily quota for protein isn't difficult.

Many adults with ADHD get off to a bad start every morning by skipping breakfast—a crucial link in the daily protein chain—or by grabbing a cup of coffee and a donut, which provide zero grams of protein and lots of sugar and fat. If you're too busy to make breakfast, consider jump-starting your day with a protein shake. You can buy protein shake mixes at the local health food store and some grocery stores. Simply toss the mix into the blender with some fruit and ice, push "pulse," and you've got an instant protein shake.

Combining Diet and Medication

You might be wondering whether there are certain foods you should avoid combining with stimulant drugs, whether you are going to lose a lot of weight, or whether you should time your meals or medication to ensure optimal effectiveness of stimulant drugs.

Foods That Interfere with Stimulant Drugs

To date, the only food you should avoid if you're taking stimulant drugs is grapefruit juice, which interferes with the way the body absorbs and breaks down amphetamines. If you take your medication in the morning before breakfast and drink grapefruit juice or eat a piece of grapefruit, you won't get the full benefit of the medication.

Stimulants and Weight Loss

While amphetamines increase your metabolism and may cause temporary weight loss when you begin taking them, most adults with ADHD who take stimulant drugs under a doctor's supervision do not shed significant pounds. In fact, most ADHD adults who lose weight after starting stimulant medications tend to put it back on within a few months.

If you're already underweight and concerned about losing more by taking stimulants, ask your physician to prescribe one that has less effect on weight. In general, methylphenidates cause less weight loss than amphetamines. Taking excessive amounts of stimulants could result in dramatic weight loss as well as serious consequences like depression, anxiety, and insomnia.

Timing Your Meals

One easy way to ensure you get the most from your medications is to time your meals according to the medication's instructions. Long-acting stimulants, including Adderall XR, Focalin XR, and Ritalin LA, are best taken on an empty stomach since high-fat foods could interfere with their absorption and prolong the amount of time they take to kick in. However, Concerta and Daytrana, two long-acting methylphenidate preparations, do not appear to have dietary-related absorption problems.

CHAPTER 14

Financial and Legal Issues

A dults with ADHD face challenges in keeping their finances in order, making the most of their health care benefits, and asserting their legal rights. Fortunately, there are many ways you can organize your life and make sure your ADHD doesn't get in the way. Being organized and taking the time to familiarize yourself with your health care policy and potential tax benefits can pay off big time in the long run.

Financial Strategies for ADHD Adults

Even non-ADHD parents have trouble keeping track of household finances, and it's no wonder. Bills and invoices seem to come from every direction and include household expenses and repairs, college and high school tuition and expenses, expenditures for clothing and goods, transportation expenses and car repairs, bills for dentists and routine physical exams, health club membership dues, and food expenses.

Keeping track of the medical expenses and medications related to adult ADHD and childhood ADHD is an overwhelming challenge, especially if you see multiple specialists or take multiple medications. Each doctor visit creates a paper trail that needs to be tracked for reimbursement and tax purposes.

Alert

Research shows that couples who fear and worry about not having enough money suffer heated arguments, disagreements, resentment, fear, and anger that contributes to separation and divorce. Studies show that couples where one or more partner has adult ADHD are twice as likely to divorce as non-ADHD couples, and squabbles over money, finances, and bill-paying head the list of complaints.

Many ADHD parents also have one or more children with the disorder who are seeing a variety of medical experts, and who may be attending special schools or classes or receiving specialized assistance in college or in the workplace.

Getting a Handle on Household Finances

Many common organizational strategies will help you keep your household finances in order. For instance, establishing a household calendar that includes deadlines for household bills can ensure that someone in the family remembers to pay them.

It's also wise to delegate the family bookkeeping to the spouse who is the most detail-oriented. If neither spouse feels up to the task, the best solution is to hire a bookkeeper.

Establishing Financial Records

From receipts and invoices to insurance claims and health insurance policies, sometimes it's essential to be able to quickly locate the right piece of paper. If you have adult ADHD, you may think you're too impulsive or hyperactive to have the patience for something as dull and boring as filing and tracing receipts.

Unfortunately, not doing so can result in losing hundreds or thousands of dollars. The good news is it doesn't take an MBA to set up an easy filing and tracking system for your family. You can do it yourself using these helpful tips.

❑ Buy an accordion folder for each category of expenses (medical, household, college, summer camp, etc.). The folders are too big for you to lose them, and because they are enclosed on three sides (unlike manila folders), they are a safe place to stash papers and invoices of all shapes and sizes without worrying about them slipping out.

❑ Label each section of the accordion for specific bills, such as doctor's visits, psychologist's visits, prescription medications, medical insurance, specialized classes for children, disability insurance, legal fees, and transportation and mileage. Every time you get a bill, whether it's a physician's invoice or a credit card slip for a medication, file it in the proper place.

❑ Remember to keep track of transportation and mileage to and from doctor's visits, as well as receipts for parking, turnpike tolls, gas, and/or mileage for tax deduction purposes.

❑ If you'd rather keep track of your expenses via computer, Quicken Medical software is an ideal organizational tool for ADHD adults. It lets you electronically file insurance information, provider information, exam histories, payments, and disputed claims for each family member in one place. The program also automatically calculates reimbursable mileage, tax deductions, and flexible spending account contributions. Visit *www.quickenmedical.com* for details.

By keeping track of medical bills, you'll save money you'd otherwise lose on erroneous credit card statements, higher interest rates and penalties, and lost insurance claims. You'll also avoid the stress and worry of wondering if you've paid a bill on time. In addition, if you feel you've been denied a legitimate insurance claim for a medical bill, you'll have copies of everything you need to fight your case and win.

Managing Costs

Paying for the diagnosis, evaluation, and treatment of adult ADHD can take a toll on your finances. Fortunately, there are tax breaks and assistance programs to help you, and your insurance company can help you cover the health care you need.

Flexible Spending Accounts

One way to get a handle on expenses is to look into a flexible spending account (FSA) if it's offered by your employer. By estimating your medical expenses, you may save lots of money throughout the year. With a flexible spending account, you set aside a certain amount of money from each paycheck before taxes and then draw on that money in your FSA for medical expenses. For more information, see IRS Publication 969 at *www .irs.gov/publications/p969*.

Tax Deductions

Be sure to research medical tax deductions, which may include everything from co-pays and diagnostic testing to transportation expenses to and from medical specialists. For a complete list of medical expenses that the IRS may count toward an FSA or medical tax deductions, see IRS Publication 502 at *www .irs.gov/publications/p502*.

Help with Medication Costs

If you're uninsured or underinsured and can't afford your medication for adult ADHD, consider looking into patient assistance programs. For a list of drug manufacturers and government and local organizations that may be able to help you get free or reduced-cost prescription drugs, visit *www.helpingpatients.com*, a website sponsored by the Pharmaceutical Research and Manufacturers of America.

Recoup Lost Money

If you've been suffering from adult ADHD for years but were only diagnosed recently, you could reclaim past medical expenses on your tax return. You have three years to file a retroactive claim, provided you kept all your receipts and a record of allowable deductions. For more information on filing an amended tax return, see IRS Publication 17, Tax Guide, at *www.irs.gov/pub/irs-pdf/p17.pdf.*

Insurance Matters

Dealing with adult ADHD can be extremely costly, especially if you have inadequate health insurance, don't understand what your insurance plan does and doesn't cover, and aren't aware of the many tax breaks and special assistance programs available to adults with ADHD.

Unfortunately, rising medical costs have led some insurance companies to deny claims, even when they're legitimate. The good news is that many states have established independent review panels and set up regulations that require insurance companies to develop in-house appeal procedures.

Essential

If your insurance company refuses to pay a claim, consider appealing. While fighting a denied claim can be a time-consuming process, studies by the Kaiser Family Foundation showed that 52 percent of patients who appealed won their first appeal, 44 percent won their second appeal, and 45 percent won the third time around.

Although many insurance companies have a limit on how much money they'll pay out per year for treatment for adult ADHD, you may be able to persuade your insurance company to pay a higher percentage of costs by documenting that your need for medical care exceeds what is offered on your policy.

Scoping Out Carriers

If you've been diagnosed recently with adult ADHD, spend some time talking with your insurance carrier to find out what portion of medical expenses you'll be responsible for. If you have a choice of carriers or plans, compare them carefully and select the one that best suits your needs and will save you the most money in the long run.

When reviewing your policy, you'll also want to check if it covers mental health benefits. Find out what types of services it covers and whether it covers outpatient and inpatient care and serious as well as nonserious diagnoses.

Fact

Unfortunately, some insurance companies don't consider adult ADHD a "serious" condition, even though it typically is. To move things along, have your physician send your provider a letter of medical necessity along with test results showing your need for treatment. Remember that insurance companies are huge bureaucracies, so keep meticulous records of who said what, and date every correspondence.

You'll also want to call your insurance company and ask about prerequisites for receiving mental health benefits, the number of visits you're permitted per year, whether multiple services can be scheduled on one day to count as one visit, and what services require pre-authorization and who needs to authorize them.

If your physicians or specialists aren't covered in your plan, you may want to explain your situation ahead of time and ask them if they can either accept your insurance plan, give you the same rate as your insurance plan, or give you discounted health care.

Finally, if the thought of dealing with insurance paperwork and hassles gives you migraines, consider hiring someone who specializes in handling insurance claims for adults with ADHD. It could be an accountant or even a financial coach. Call your local branch of CHADD for suggestions on accountants who work with people with ADHD, ask members of your support group for suggestions, or work with a trained coach who specializes in adult ADHD by contacting the International Coach Federation at (888) 423-3131 or by visiting *www.coachfederation.org*.

Your specialist can file and keep track of claims, follow up on payments and claims discrepancies, negotiate rates with your medical specialists, and ensure you get the best health care for your money.

Diagnoses and Legalities

If you've just been diagnosed with adult ADHD, you're probably wondering who to tell and how much to say. Many adults with ADHD are worried their employer can demote them, lower their salary, or even fire them if they find out about their disability. Others wonder if it's worth divulging their disability to receive special services and compensations. Although it comes down to a personal decision, here is some general advice.

Should I Tell My Boss?

There's no law saying you have to tell your employer you have adult ADHD. In fact, it's against the law for your employer to ask you questions about your medical or psychiatric history. It's also illegal for your employer to demote you, lower your salary, or fire you in the event he discovers you have adult ADHD.

If you feel you've been discriminated against for having adult ADHD, your best recourse is to contact the U.S. Equal Employment Opportunity Commission (*www.eeoc.gov*) within 180 days of the alleged discrimination. (Note that some state or local laws provide additional time on the basis of a disability, so research the laws that apply in your area.)

The Ins and Outs of the ADA

The Americans with Disabilities Act (ADA) was established by Congress in 1990 to end discrimination in the workplace and to provide equal employment opportunities for people with disabilities, including children and adults with ADHD. The ADA applies to all businesses with fifteen or more employees, including private employers, state and local governments, employment agencies, labor organizations, and labor-management committees.

Am I Eligible for ADA Coverage?

Although the ADA covers mental conditions and illnesses, including adult ADHD, getting a diagnosis for the condition will not automatically qualify you for protection. To do so, you must show that your condition imposes significant limitations on a major life activity or function. You must also be regarded as having a disability, have a record of having been viewed as being disabled, and be able to perform the essential job functions with or without accommodations.

In order to be covered by the ADA, you must tell your employer you have adult ADHD. If your employer doesn't know you have a disability or how it could affect your job performance, he wouldn't be able to provide services to help you do your job. This is especially true if you accepted a job and signed a written job description that described duties you knew would pose difficulties for you, such as organizing projects, turning things in on time, and working well with others.

If you qualify for the ADA, your employer is required by law to make accommodations for you unless he can prove that making these accommodations would create an undue hardship to the company in terms of expense, time, and logistics.

Accommodations could include restructuring your job duties, adjusting your schedule or hours, reassigning you to a more appropriate position, or modifying testing and training materials and policy manuals.

Am I Eligible for Social Security Benefits?

If you have adult ADHD, you may qualify for Social Security Disability Insurance or disability benefits from Supplemental Security Income (SSI). Like anyone applying for SSI, you must first receive a medical determination that will review your attention problems, medical history, and the limitations the condition puts on your ability to function and make a living.

Alert

If you were diagnosed with childhood ADHD and qualified for Social Security Disability Insurance under Social Security Administration (SSA) regulations, the SSA will review your case when you turn eighteen to determine if you qualify for benefits under the adult regulations. Even if your condition has not improved, your benefits will stop if you don't meet the adult criteria.

If you can document that you haven't been able to engage in work above the monthly substantial gainful work activity limit for the past twelve months because of adult ADHD, or you anticipate you won't be able to engage in such work for twelve months, there's a chance you may be entitled to Social Security benefits.

Diagnosis for Legal Reasons

If you need a lawyer to help you sort through employment issues related to your adult ADHD, make sure you hire an attorney who specializes in helping people who have the condition.

As a general rule of thumb, you may want to consider hiring a lawyer in these scenarios:

❏ The facts are simple and easily established, and you believe you have a clear-cut case of discrimination, wrongful firing, etc.

❏ The results of losing your job would be catastrophic and pose severe financial hardships.

❏ The amount of money and time you'd have to spend on litigation fees won't exceed the amount of money you believe you're due.

❏ You've tried and failed to settle or resolve the issue outside of court.

❏ Your claim for special assistance has been rejected.

For more information about your legal rights as an adult with ADHD and associated learning disabilities, visit the National Center for Learning Disabilities at *www.ncld.org*. For the name of a good adult ADHD lawyer, ask for recommendations from members of your support group or local disability organizations. You may also want to contact state and local chapters of Children and Adults with Attention Deficit/Hyperactivity Disorder (CHADD; *www.chadd.org*).

CHAPTER 15

Making Necessary
Lifestyle Changes

Many ADHD adults struggle to overcome years of guilt and shame stemming from negative behavior patterns and attitudes they assumed were personal flaws. If you've just been diagnosed with adult ADHD, the good news is it's never too late to learn how to manage your symptoms and make the most of the special gifts that come along with adult ADHD, like harnessing your energy and enthusiasm for a new career that matches your talents and temperament.

Changing Negative Beliefs and Attitudes

As many great thinkers have attested over the centuries, external changes start on the inside. Before you can make positive changes that impact your talents, your relationships, your job, and your physical health, you need to change the way you think about and view yourself. When you have a disorder like adult ADHD that comes with so many built-in negatives, one effective way to begin to change the way you perceive yourself is to look at the positive side of your ADHD traits.

The Bright Side of Hyperactivity
Many adults with ADHD have turned their natural hyperactivity into an asset by tapping into their bottomless reservoir of energy

to help them accomplish more in one day that most people can accomplish in a week. Some of the world's most accomplished artists, writers, painters, inventors, politicians, and filmmakers have harnessed their hyperactivity and turned it into fame and fortune.

Like them, you can reframe negative ADHD characteristics into positives that can help you achieve your wildest dreams. Here are some examples of new ways to look at adult ADHD symptoms.

- I have so much more energy that other people that I can get projects done long before they're due and still have time for the things I enjoy doing.
- Because I have the energy and stamina to accomplish more than most people, I can use it to learn more, get ahead faster, and use my knowledge to achieve great things.
- Because I'm very busy and productive, I burn up a lot of mental and physical energy every day and am usually able to get a good night's sleep.
- The more experience I have, the more information I have about what I really love to do, what I do well, and what type of things I merely tolerate.

Inattention

While adult ADHD is a disorder that involves a lack of attention, for many adults, the problem is that they pay too much attention to things that interest them and ignore everything else.

Fact

Some adults with ADHD are highly intuitive and able to pick up on unexpressed emotion, subtle body language, and nonverbal communication, although many others have enormous difficulty reading nonverbal cues. This may explain why a disproportionate number of psychologists and psychiatrists are ADHD adults—and a good example of how you can turn an adult ADHD negative into a positive.

The hyperfocus of adult ADHD is what allowed an inventor like Guglielmo Marconi to develop the wireless telegraph. He was able to get up every day, focus on his fledging invention, and blank out everything else—including his financial, health, and marital problems. Here are some ways to change your negative perceptions regarding inattention.

- Maybe the reason I'm not paying attention is because I'm bored with this job and I need to think about searching for a job that will fully utilize my talents.
- I know other people need to read the entire manual to figure out how to do this, but maybe I should respect the fact that I already understand how to do this without having to slog through the fine print.
- I'm not really interested in going go the opera with my wife, but maybe if I opened myself up to the idea, I would learn something new and enjoyable or find a new way to relax with my wife that would improve our marriage.
- I'm very lucky that I was able to hyperfocus on the tiny details that made this project so successful. This is a quality I can use to do superior work in every aspect of my life.

Distractibility

There's a silver lining to being easily distracted if you work in life-and-death situations like emergency medical care or firefighting. For instance, firefighters are often able to detect smoke before others and can react quickly.

Medical experts often notice small details that may have been overlooked by others—such as a small change in the color of a mole, or a lump that looks suspicious. Their internal early warning system enables them to save lives before symptoms become so serious the condition is irreversible.

Essential

On the hit TV series *House*, Dr. House is easily distracted by unusual stimuli. Because he is able to make lightning-speed associations between seemingly unrelated medical problems or symptoms, he arrives at "out of the blue" diagnoses that are nearly always correct, which amazes his colleagues.

If you suffer from distractibility, try looking for ways to flip it from a negative to a positive attribute. Here are some examples.

- I'm really glad I noticed that new little mole on my leg and went to see a dermatologist before it became any bigger.
- My husband always kids me about my overly refined sense of smell and says I really don't need to wash his jeans every single night for them to smell clean. But if I hadn't smelled what I thought was natural gas in the kitchen, our house may have burned down before the fire department was able to get here.
- People at work told me I was just paranoid when I told them I had a horrible feeling about our new boss. Sure enough, two months later, she fired everyone in the department and replaced them with people from her old firm. If I hadn't trusted my gut feelings and found another job before this happened, I'd be out of work like my former colleagues.

Impulsivity

While impulsivity can be a dangerous trait if it propels you to do something reckless, careless, and stupid, it also means you're more willing to take leaps of faith that would leave less courageous types shaking in their boots. The history books are full of famous ADHD inventors, entrepreneurs, and artists who went out on a limb to forge new ways of doing things and left more cautious colleagues in the dust. Without all those impulsive ADHD inventors throughout history, we might still be traveling in stagecoaches or using quill pens to write reports. If you always seem to be ahead of the curve when it comes to anything new, you may be "suffering" from impulsivity. Here are some examples of how to turn it to your advantage.

- I'm really glad my impulsivity prompted me to accept a new position I wasn't sure I'd succeed at. Now I'm making a lot more money and doing work that is much more stimulating and rewarding.
- I was pretty nervous about asking one particular woman out after seeing her once at the coffee shop, but my instincts told me to go for it, so I picked up the phone and called her. If I hadn't called her, we probably never would have met again. Making that first scary phone call resulted in a happy marriage and four beautiful kids!
- I know a lot of people probably think rock climbing is risky. But after learning the techniques, I'm able to climb in a way that minimizes danger but still exposes me to the adrenaline rush I crave.

Three Easy Steps from Negatives to Positive

Overcoming the negative aspects of ADHD is a step-by-step process of exploring your negative behaviors for ways they can be turned around to your benefit. Here are three easy steps to get you from negative to positive using impulsivity as an example.

1. Understand how you are reacting to your symptoms. Realize your symptoms—not you—are in control and are actively preventing you from getting where you want to go. If your impulsivity always lands you in hot water, that's a pretty good sign you're not harnessing your impulsivity in a positive way.

2. Brainstorm how you can make lemonade from lemons. Thinking outside the box (something you already excel at), write down a list of things you can do with your impulsivity that would actually benefit you at home, at work, with your family, with friends, and in social settings.

3. Make one change at a time. Start closing the gap between negative and positive by working on one strategy to gradually change a negative trait into a positive one. For instance, if your impulsivity led you down a ski slope you didn't have the moves to master, find another area of life where you can take a risk that won't land you in the emergency ward. It could be creating a more efficient, easier, or inexpensive way to do something at work, or using your impulsivity to propel yourself into a new career that others might not have the courage to attempt.

As a person with ADHD, you have some disadvantages that simply need to be thought of as advantages—kind of like building a door to knock on when one isn't there. The key to success is to gradually transform negative, unproductive thoughts and feelings into more positive, productive behaviors that get better results and turn your liabilities into assets.

Setting and Meeting Realistic Goals

Whether you want to set a goal for losing weight, developing better eating habits, or accomplishing a project at work, it's important to have a game plan that spells out how you plan to proceed.

Keep It Specific

Whatever you want to accomplish, make your goal as specific and explicit as possible. State exactly what you want to accomplish and then determine a reasonable timeline for meeting your goal.

The simple fact is that if you don't set goals, you won't achieve them. To get the ball rolling, commit to your goal in writing and write down a realistic deadline for completing the goal. Be sure to break the goal down into small, doable, bit-by-bit steps.

Track Your Goals

To keep yourself on schedule, make sure your goal is something you can track during each step. Avoid nebulous goals that can't be measured.

If your goal is to lose ten pounds in a month, weigh yourself every day and track your progress on a weight calendar and includes notes to yourself about what worked, what didn't work, and any setbacks. It may also help to record your thoughts and emotions in a weight-loss diary so you can avoid thought patterns that lead to overeating and bingeing.

Make Sure Your Goals Are Realistic for You

Set realistic goals that you actually have a good chance of accomplishing, rather than pie-in-the-sky goals that set you up for failure. Again, an important point is to take one small, doable step in the right direction at a time.

Essential

If you want to lose weight, don't set yourself up for failure by setting a goal of losing twenty-five pounds in one month. Very few people can lose that much weight in four weeks without inviting serious health risks.

Also, remember that setting goals you know are impossible is just another way of not setting a goal at all. Sooner or later, you'll be forced to tell yourself that it's okay to bag the goal, because the truth is you never could have accomplished it anyway.

Make Sure Your Goals Are Relevant

Your goals have to be important to you, and they also have to be goals you think are worthy of accomplishing for them to yield fruit. You're not going to lose weight, earn more money, or organize your office just because your wife or boss tells you that you should. To be meaningful to you, your goals have to start from the inside. Don't let anyone bully you and set goals for you that you aren't ready, willing, or able to accomplish.

Give Yourself a Realistic Deadline

Telling yourself you're going to lose weight "when the mood hits me" or "when I have more time to exercise" is a recipe for failure. To give your goals legs, set a realistic deadline with measurable benchmarks along the way that give you a sense of accomplishment and optimism.

Let's say your goal is to research and write a report in one month. Divide the goal up into smaller tasks and assign each task a due date. Put deadlines for each task on a calendar, along with reminder notes that the task is due in a week, three days, two days, or one hour. Then cross off each task as you complete it so you have a visual record of your progress.

Learning Stress Management

Sitting in a miles-long traffic jam, losing an important file, or missing a flight can rattle anyone's sense of composure, but for ADHD adults, stressful situations have a tendency to spiral into disasters because of the twin ADHD symptoms of impatience and impulsivity.

By learning some simple stress-management techniques, you can prevent what could be a devastating and destructive chain of events from ever happening.

Take Deep Breaths

Start by taking ten—breaths, that is. The simple action of inhaling and exhaling ten times will redirect your focus from that missed plane to your bodily rhythms (you're still alive and breathing, so what else matters?), give you some literal "breathing space" to collect your thoughts, and give your temper a chance to cool down.

Move It or Lose It

Another way to shake off stress is to exercise or move. Exercise releases hormones that make you feel more content and happy. If you can't squeeze in a workout, take a few minutes to stretch, move your shoulders, scrunch your face, or take a quick walk outdoors. Exposing yourself to sunlight will also help alleviate a funk.

Beep and Buzz Yourself

If you're stressed out because you lost track of time and blew a deadline, set your watch or cell phone to beep or buzz at regular intervals to remind you to stay on track.

Just Say No

ADHD adults have a bad habit of promising more than they can deliver, so resist your natural tendency to say yes to every request. Know when to say no. It's better to turn down a project you know you can't handle than to sabotage yourself by promising to do it, failing to deliver, and stressing over it all the while.

Send Negative Thoughts Packing

Practice mentally removing yourself from stress-producing thoughts or actions so those thoughts are no longer your problems.

Prepare for Automatic Pilot

To prevent stress from happening in the first place, figure out logistical steps and strategies that can help keep stress at bay. For instance, if you never seem to get to work on time, put everything out the night before so you don't have to think when you wake up the next morning. Lay out your clothing, have your box of cereal and fruit handy, set your briefcase or laptop by the door, and fill your gas tank the night before.

Stop the Blame Game

Blaming yourself for symptoms caused by a neurobiological imbalance is like blaming yourself for being born with brown eyes instead of blue. If you can't seem to shake your feelings of guilt, you may want to try cognitive behavioral therapy, which helps you shift the blame from yourself to your adult ADHD.

For additional support, join a local ADHD support group or hook into an online network of people who can support you. You'll discover even more ideas and get positive solutions that can help.

Get Adequate Sleep

Studies show that up to 70 percent of ADHD adults have trouble falling asleep, staying asleep, and getting enough sleep. If getting enough shut-eye sometimes seems like a daydream that will never happen to you, you may need to establish better sleep habits.

 Alert

Recent studies have isolated four distinct reasons to explain why ADHD adults have impaired sleep habits and often find themselves wide awake at 3 A.M., when they long to be in dreamland, and dead tired at 3 P.M., when they are nodding off at their desk.

As an ADHD adult, it's important not to blame yourself for insomnia or daytime drowsiness. The fact is that you're far more prone to sleep disturbances than other people because of your innate mental and physical restlessness, hyperactivity, impulsivity, and impatience. If you take stimulant medications that increase your metabolism and heart rate, you may be at an even higher risk of developing sleep problems.

Night Owls

About 75 percent of ADHD adults have trouble quieting their racing minds when it's time to hunker down and fall asleep. Some are self-described night owls who don't really feel alive until the sun goes down, while others find it impossible to "turn off" their brains and racing thoughts, even if they've been tired all day and been looking forward to going to sleep. Research shows that more than 70 percent of ADHD adults spend more than an hour every night trying to fall asleep.

Princess and the Pea Sleepers

For some ADHD adults, the problem isn't falling asleep but the quality of sleep. They may toss and turn all night, wake up frequently, or be disturbed by a partner's movements or snoring.

Sleep of the Dead

Some experts report more than 80 percent of ADHD adults wake up over and over throughout the night before falling into such a deep sleep that they can't even be roused by multiple alarm clocks, blinding daylight, or rigorous shaking by family members. Difficult wakers are often extremely moody and grouchy when forcibly awakened.

Asleep on Your Feet

One theory holds that when some ADHD adults become disinterested or bored with something, their normal hyperfocus switch abruptly turns off. Their nervous system disengages so they become extremely sleepy. They may even nod off into what is called "intrusive sleep," a sleep that interrupts life when you least expect it.

Of course, the snooze-and-crash syndrome is especially dangerous if you happen to be driving when it occurs. Research shows that long-distance driving on straight, monotonous roads induces intrusive sleep.

If you've been diagnosed with this condition, it's important to plan ahead so you don't become a moving hazard. If you have a business trip that entails night driving, bring someone else along who can take over the wheel when the sun goes down. If you're planning a family vacation on the road, consider arranging the itinerary so you can do most of the driving during the day, or let your wife do the driving at night.

Second Wind

Many ADHD adults seem to get a surge of energy and sense of purpose right around the time everyone else is going to sleep. After a long day of feeling disorganized and spaced out, it may feel natural to simply go with your natural impulse to stay up late and capitalize on your "night owl" nature.

 Alert

Sleeping in late on Sunday and getting up early on Monday morning will create the equivalent of jet lag in your body, and is likely to leave you feeling groggy and unable to concentrate. To wake up feeling alert during the work week, get up on weekends at the same time you get up for work.

Experts believe you're better off trying to establish a normal sleep cycle so your work hours jive with the rest of the working world.

If you're currently going to bed at 3 A.M., try moving your bed-time back by 15 minutes every week until you're hitting the sack at a more desirable hour. Set the mood for sleep by removing distractions from your bedroom and avoiding rigorous exercise and large meals right before bedtime.

Many people find that reading something light, comforting, dry, or technical helps clear their mind and induce sleep. Others find listening to classical music, jazz, or inspirational tapes helpful. If, like many ADHD adults, you find that you have your most creative ideas at night, keep a notepad and pen by the bed and write them down.

Establish Good Eating Habits

Many people with adult ADHD function most effectively on a high-protein diet that is low in simple sugars and carbohydrates.

The Role of Essential Fatty Acids

Foods high in essential fatty acids, including omega-6 and omega-3, have been shown to promote brain functioning. Because your body doesn't manufacture these acids, it's important to eat foods that provide them.

Foods high in essential fatty acids include fruits; whole grains; cold-water fish like salmon, tuna, and sardines; seeds like flax, sesame, and pumpkin; nuts like walnuts and brazil nuts; avocados; dark leafy vegetables like spinach, kale, and mustard greens; and healthy cold-pressed oils like canola, olive oil, soybean oil, and wheat germ oil.

Eliminating Sugar Crashes

Foods high in simple sugars and carbohydrates run the gamut from candy, cake, and junk food to white flour, pasta, potatoes, corn, white rice, and other unrefined foods.

 Fact

Consider pairing a sweet treat, potato, or bowl of rice with a portion of protein to stabilize your blood sugar levels. This can help you ward off hyperactivity and inattention that may be triggered by sugar highs, and moodiness, depression, irritability, and lethargy caused by sugar lows.

As an ADHD adult, you're probably already struggling with inattention, an inability to pay attention and focus, and scattered thinking. Overloading on simple sugars may exacerbate existing problems and send you into sugar overload. In addition, just as some ADHD adults are hypersensitive to loud noises, others are hypersensitive to the taste, smell, and texture of specific foods.

If you can't figure out what to eat or avoid, or if you are having trouble eating a balanced diet because of an aversion to certain foods, you may want to consult a nutritionist or registered dietitian who is familiar with adult ADHD. She can help you develop a meal plan and recipes that satisfy your hunger and cravings for your favorite foods and eliminate those foods that exacerbate symptoms.

Get Regular Exercise

While research is limited, it's clear that regular exercise decreases depression in adults with ADHD, improves your ability to handle stress, and may even cause small improvements in memory and learning. If you're new to exercise or if your ADHD symptoms have made it increasingly difficult for you to get back to exercising, here are some helpful tricks that may help you get back on the treadmill.

❑ Exercise before going to work. A hectic day or changes in schedule can squeeze out time for exercise later in the day, so do it first thing in the morning. Most people do their best creative thinking during or after a workout, so you'll also be bringing your best brain to work with you.

❑ Just do it. If you wake up feeling groggy or tired, don't use it as an excuse to avoid exercising. Just start exercising anyhow, and you'll probably find that your drowsiness vanishes in moments and you end your workout feeling more energized than before you started.

❏ Keep it simple. Do regular exercise that meshes with your schedule and lifestyle. If you live near the ocean, try walking or running on the beach. If you live in the mountains, use the hills as your personal stair-climbing machine. If your exercise routine entails driving to a health club that is a half hour away, there's a good chance you'll find lots of excuses to avoid it.

❏ Keep it playful. There's no need to turn your exercise workout into a grunt-like boot camp. Choose activities you enjoy and you'll be more likely to stick with your program. If you get bored easily, schedule a different activity for every day of your workout to keep things interesting. For example, walk on Mondays, bicycle on Wednesdays, hit the treadmill on Fridays, and hike on Sundays.

❏ Don't mistake mental fatigue for physical fatigue. If you work out during the day or after work, you may sometimes feel too "brain-fogged" to think about tying on your running shoes. Instead of telling yourself you're too exhausted to exercise, agree that you'll do ten minutes of your workout, and if you still feel tired, call it quits. Most likely, before your ten minutes are up, you'll feel so awake and energized that you won't even be tempted to stop.

❏ Don't be a slave to your workout. You should exercise enough to maintain toned muscles and a healthy heart—but not so much that you risk overuse syndrome or injuries. Exercising for thirty minutes three to four times a week is enough to get and keep you in good shape. You can do longer activities, but remember that moderation is key.

Getting a Handle on Clutter

Clutter may be one of your worst enemies. It wastes time and energy because it prevents you from getting organized, finding things, and meeting deadlines.

☐ Essential

Clutter prevents you from seeing the big picture so you can break it down into smaller, doable tasks. When your entire life is full of clutter, all you can see are millions of disorganized and seemingly unrelated pieces of a larger puzzle that you'd love to assemble but don't know where to start.

As family members or roommates would probably admit, clutter can also make you difficult to live with, primarily because your clutter has no limits and often infringes on other people's space. Before they can get anything done, they have to deal with your clutter first, too.

The Problem with Perfection

According to ADHD experts, the biggest reason many ADHD adults don't make a dent in their clutter is because they are afraid they won't be able to de-clutter 100 percent and wind up with an ultra-organized home.

Remember two important things when it comes to de-cluttering your environment. Every journey begins with a single step, and making small changes can result in major improvements. For instance, think of how easy it would be to find two socks that match every morning if you simply rolled matching pairs of socks together when they came out of the dryer instead of stuffing them into your drawer.

Implementing Organization and Structure

If you're gazing out over a sea of your personal clutter, you've probably become rather defensive about what people living with you may regard as your personal pigsty. Clutter doesn't have to sabotage your relationships, your career, or your life. Here are seven simple ways to eliminate clutter and bring more organization and structure to your life.

1. Start with the most important room of your life. Focus on the area of your life that would most benefit from de-cluttering and begin there. If it's your job, start with your office. If your clutter has made it impossible for your wife to cook meals, begin in the kitchen. Don't get bogged down with miscellaneous considerations, whether it's time, convenience, aesthetics, practicality, or money.

2. Keep it simple. Make a list of no more than five tasks you want to complete first. Cross off each task as you complete it to give yourself a sense of accomplishment.

3. Find a clutter buddy. Find a friend or family member willing to keep you from giving up on clutter as you tackle what is likely to feel utterly boring. Your clutter buddy should not help you de-clutter, but should set the tone by doing something productive but unrelated to your task.

4. Guard against hyperfocus. Limit your de-cluttering activities to a set time period, then stop for the day. Set an alarm to signal it's time to stop. If you keep your de-cluttering sessions short, you won't wear yourself out the first time, which may discourage you from getting back to it.

5. Make filing fun. Create a filing system so you can find things the next time you need them. One easy way to do this is to by a pre-made filing system from the Container Store (*www.containerstore.com*) called File Solutions, which comes with color-coded sections, preprinted labels, and a directory of where to put things.

6. Buy a paper shredder. Looking at a mountain of paper clutter and wondering if it's safe to just heave it in the trash? With the growing frequency of identity theft, a thief could wipe out your bank account using a credit card slip duplicate you forgot to file. Play it safe and shred any

receipts or documents that might contain personal information such as credit card numbers, Social Security numbers, driver's licenses, birthdays, and personal ID numbers. If you get a lot of junk mail, put the paper shredder next to the trash can so you can feed unwanted flyers and brochures into it before they have a chance to become clutter on your desk.

7. Turn your trash into treasure. If your de-cluttering efforts have left you with piles of stuff that are worthless to you but too valuable to throw away or donate to Goodwill, hold a yard sale and watch your trash turn into cold hard cash.

There's a larger silver lining to de-cluttering. Once you've flattened your piles, cleared away the heaps of junk, and actually made money getting rid of your clutter, you'll feel a new sense of control over yourself and your life, and you'll be far less likely to clutter it up again.

CHAPTER 16

Coping with Adult ADHD in Social Settings

As an adult member of society, you're expected to interact and communicate with others on a regular basis, be capable of understanding what people say, and be able to read and interpret nonverbal cues so you can behave appropriately. Unfortunately, many ADHD adults can't follow conversations, stay focused on lengthy discussions, or read nonverbal cues or body language. Because they exist in an information vacuum, they often respond to conversations or social interactions in ways that are not appropriate, consistent, or relevant.

Symptoms That Flare in Social Settings

It's not unusual to experience these common adult ADHD symptoms that tend to flare up in social settings:

- Feeling like you don't fit in
- Having trouble following conversations
- Having difficulty zoning out extraneous noises or music
- Feeling overwhelmed
- Feeling the need to dominate a conversation
- Blurting out confidential, inappropriate, or irrelevant information during conversations

- Being unable to read and translate body language, voice tone, facial expressions, or simple nuances of interaction
- Reacting in an overemotional, defensive, or overly intense way
- Jumping to the wrong conclusions
- Feeling defensive
- Feeling that others are criticizing and blaming you
- Being reluctant to contribute or participate in a conversation because you're afraid of embarrassing yourself
- Being viewed by others as standoffish, disinterested, snobbish, or bored

Practice Makes Perfect

Before going to a party, try rehearsing some responses to questions that typically arise in casual party chat. Standard questions you might be asked include "What do you do for a living?" or "What do you do for fun or to relax?" Try practicing your responses with an understanding friend, spouse, or therapist, in various fictional settings. For example, imagine what you'd say to someone at the buffet table, at the bar, around a formal dinner table, in a friend's kitchen, by the pool, around the barbecue, or while playing croquet.

Go to Social Functions with a Party Buddy

Instead of trying to weather a social function on your own, ask a close friend to go with you. You'll have someone on hand to translate conversations you have trouble following, interpret nonverbal cues, and give you a friendly nudge or warning look when you start to stray.

Your buddy can also test the waters of small groups at a party by joining the conversation first. If it seems like a friendly group and a conversation you'll be able to participate in successfully, he can wave you in and introduce you.

Listen Before Speaking

Before jumping into a conversation, listen for several minutes to make sure you fully understand what is being discussed. Collect your thoughts, quiet your mind, and think about what you could say that would add to the conversation.

Bow Out Before Blowing Out

If you find yourself in a small group discussion you either can't follow or can't keep up with, don't wrack your brain trying to think up an appropriate response that may not hit the mark.

If you're truly confused and/or bewildered by the train of conversation, or if the topic of conversation is simply over your head, find a good excuse to bow out politely before you've reached the point of no return, when your hyperactivity or impulsivity causes you to butt in or blurt out something that may be inappropriate or irrelevant. "Where's the restroom?" or "I'd better rejoin my friend," or "I think I need a glass of water" are a few good excuses.

L. Essential

One effective way to bond with someone you've just met is to model their body language. If they cross your arms, you cross your arms. If they use hand gestures when talking, you do the same. The trick is to be subtle. If you're too obvious about modeling, the other person may mistake it for ridicule or mockery and become insulted.

Match the Tone of the Conversation

If the tone of conversation is silly and funny, don't respond with serious or heavy comments, or the conversation may stop dead. Or, if you're in a group that's discussing death or a serious topic, be respectful and solemn in turn instead of chiming in with a flippant or sarcastic comment.

If you're listening to a conversation about politics, religion, or a controversial topic and someone says something you vehemently disagree with, don't feel compelled to argue or make your point unless you're openly encouraged to by other members of the group.

Essential

> If you sense you're seriously outnumbered in your opinion about something, it may be best to keep your thoughts to yourself. Unless you're an excellent debater and can argue your point without getting defensive, combative, argumentative, or flustered, you're better off not starting a heated argument that could force you to lose your cool or your temper.

If you feel like it's a good idea to try to argue your point, make sure you have your facts straight, then state your case briefly and politely—and with a smile to show you're not trying to convert anyone or start a fight. Remember that unless you're at a political rally, a party is not the place or time to get on your political soap box.

Be Upbeat, Not Negative

Before heading off to a party, remind yourself of the strengths you have that will make you enjoyable to be with and talk with. Maybe you're very generous, are a great mimic, or have a wonderful sense of humor. Embracing your gifts will help others see them.

Limit Your Personal Disclosure

Don't let your impulsivity or hyperactivity lead you to share too much about yourself with strangers or people you don't know very well. This could make them feel uncomfortable and pressured to reciprocate with personal details about themselves.

For instance, does a casual new acquaintance really want to hear all the gruesome details that led to your recent divorce? Do you really want to share the gory details of your bypass surgery with total strangers?

 Fact

> While it may be tempting to turn yourself into the center of attention for a few moments by spilling your guts, remember that sharing too much personal information with casual strangers may cast you in a negative or less-than-favorable light. People who don't know you well won't have enough positive information to balance out the negative input you're giving them.

There's also the risk that sharing too much overly positive information about yourself could come across as bragging or boasting. There's also a chance that some people might be left wondering if you're telling the truth, or simply exaggerating or lying to try to impress or intimidate them.

Sharing too much about yourself with casual acquaintances could have the opposite effect you were hoping to achieve. Instead of making people feel closer to you, it could send them running in the opposite direction and leave you feeling alone and isolated.

Don't Hog the Conversation

Because they have trouble reading nonverbal cues, many ADHD adults have a tendency to dominate conversations or keep talking long after everyone has lost interest.

If you're talking with a group of people, try to listen far more than you talk, and keep your comments short, kind, and honest (but not overly blunt). Also, be careful not to jump into conversations before you're invited, and limit your comments to the topic at hand rather than dominating the conversation with irrelevant or unrelated matters.

How to Master Small Talk

Even if you're an expert in your field and can converse for hours at a time on specific intellectual issues, if you have adult ADHD there's a good chance you find it difficult to engage in the sort of chit chat and small talk that is common at social gatherings. This is especially true if the conversation is about something you're not familiar with.

One of the easiest ways to make small talk is practice asking preset questions that can be used in a variety of conversations. For instance, you can tell someone you really like a part of their outfit and ask them who made it, where they found it, what is it made of, etc.

Another easy way to facilitate small talk is to read up on local and international news before going to a party so you have lots of easy conversation starters at your disposal.

Dealing with Anger

Many ADHD adults are easily annoyed and frustrated, and are known for angry outbursts. If this sounds familiar, it's important to realize you don't have to be held captive by a short temper. By mastering some easy strategies, you can gain the upper hand on your temperamental nature.

- ❏ List your triggers. Write a list of scenarios, situations, and people that test your patience or make you lose your cool. Then practice responding to trigger points by counting to ten, taking deep breaths, or visualizing yourself neutralizing the comment or situation so it no longer angers you.
- ❏ Take the long view. Count to ten and consider the chain of events your angry reaction would trigger as opposed to what would happen if you responded calmly.
- ❏ Be angry before you reset. Instead of reacting immediately to a bad situation, give yourself permission to be angry for a set amount of time, say five or ten minutes. Then put the

angry thought out of your head and move on to something else. Stewing and fuming for extended periods of time will fuel the flames and turn a bonfire into a forest fire.

❑ Distract yourself from anger. If a critical coworker blames you for a mistake you didn't make, instead of lashing back, pull out a photo of someone who loves and admires you and remind yourself that your coworker's opinions aren't all that important to your overall happiness and well-being.

❑ Brainstorm alternate solutions to problems. As an ADHD adult, you're already a natural at brainstorming and thinking outside the box, so use your natural strengths in these areas to figure out creative solutions to problems that anger you or set you off. Create several different solutions for each problem so you can simply go on to another possible solution if one doesn't work.

❑ Look for the lighter side. When something goes wrong, reframe the situation so it becomes funny or ridiculous. Then laugh it off!

❑ Work out your anger and anxiety. If you feel your temper is nearing the end of its fuse, use exercise to extinguish the spark. Take a walk around the block, do some pushups, or take an inspiring hike or bicycle ride through nature. The feel-good endorphins exercise releases will also help ease stress and anxiety, which will help you put the situation in perspective.

❑ Talk it out with someone safe. Instead of reacting or keeping your anger bottled up inside where it's likely to fester, get it out of your system by talking it over with a nonjudgmental, supportive friend who is a good listener and can offer you sound advice.

❑ Learn to stick up for yourself. Defending yourself will make you feel less helpless and powerless—feelings that can cause you to lash out or be defensive.

How to Deal with Criticism

Many ADHD adults are understandably defensive when it comes to criticism, having endured years of it for ADHD symptoms they couldn't help or prevent. Even if the criticism was constructive or valid, or if it presented an opportunity for them to correct mistakes, they may have felt it was just another instance of someone dumping on them for something they couldn't help doing or saying, or for failing to do something they couldn't realistically accomplish.

If you tend to react negatively to all criticism, regardless of its merit, you may be missing a golden opportunity to learn and grow. Instead of automatically assuming the criticism is invalid, take a moment to really listen to what the other person is saying.

Handling Accurate Criticism

If you think there may be some truth in the criticism, ask the person making the comments to provide you with some specific examples of what he's criticizing so you can actually see what he means.

If it turns out the criticism is valid, thank the person for his suggestions and try to incorporate them next time. Instead of focusing on the mistake and criticism, shift your focus to how you can learn from it and improve.

Learning to Focus

It's difficult for ADHD adults to focus and pay attention. Because ADHD adults are easily bored when things become dull and routine, their minds tend to wander. While medication and therapy may help improve your ability to focus, you can also learn some strategies that will help you become a better and more careful listener, which in turn will help you stay connected to the conversation at hand.

Reining in a Wandering Mind

If you notice your thoughts are wandering when someone is speaking, look them in the eyes and ask them to repeat what they said, telling them that you don't want to misunderstand or misinterpret what they mean. Then repeat what they said to yourself to anchor it in your mind, keeping your eyes focused on the speaker's face.

Dismissing Distraction

If you find yourself reacting to something that's been said during a lecture and focusing more on your emotions than the content being relayed, acknowledge your emotions quickly, then temporarily dismiss them and return your attention to the speaker. Give yourself permission to re-examine your reaction to the statement after the lecture is over.

ADHD adults often find it difficult to concentrate when there is noise or music in the background. If possible, use headsets or a white noise machine to block out the noise so you can pay attention.

Doodle Your Way to Focus

If your mind is wandering during a long conversation or lecture, pick up a pen and start doodling to stay focused. Research shows it helps people pay attention. Other things that may help keep you anchored in the present include fidgeting moves like wiggling your fingers or toes, clenching your jaw, or "playing the piano" with your fingers.

Reading Nonverbal Cues

Whether it's a shoulder shrug, rolled eyes, or a hand gesture, research on nonverbal behavior tells us that what people don't say is often more important than what they do say. Unfortunately, many ADHD adults simply aren't hard-wired in a way that allows them to read or recognize nonverbal cues, interpret body language, or translate facial expressions.

Words alone often don't convey the full picture, so nonverbal behavior can either reinforce what was said or completely contradict it. An inability to read nonverbal cues and behavior can result in regular misunderstandings and confusion for many ADHD adults who are unable to recognize nonverbal cues.

Fortunately, research now shows that it's possible for ADHD adults to improve their nonverbal sensitivity by learning and practicing some specific techniques.

Look for Clues to Misunderstanding

One of the easiest ways to determine you've misunderstood something or failed to read someone's nonverbal cues is to closely analyze their behavior. Let's say you took your wife out to dinner at a fancy restaurant and before the first course arrived, you informed her she looked fat in her dress.

Fact

Even if you have trouble reading nonverbal cues, it wouldn't take a Sherlock Holmes to figure out that your wife's unusual behavior was an indication your comment had hurt or offended her. By paying close attention to how people physically or emotionally react to your behavior or comments, you can avoid making the same mistakes again.

Although your wife didn't argue with you because she knew she had, in fact, gained some weight, this doesn't mean she didn't react at all. Instead of responding verbally, she responded nonverbally by moving her chair farther away from yours, crossing her arms in front of her chest, and refusing to make eye contact with you when you spoke to her.

If you're not sure what she's feeling, learning to pay closer attention to tell-tale physical clues can help you translate non-verbal messages. For instance, you can tell she's hurt if she has angry-looking eyes, a clenched jaw, tight lips, clenched fists, or a reddened complexion. She may also physically distance herself from you by crossing her arms or legs, moving or leaning away, or giving you the cold shoulder in bed.

Rewind the Tape

If you're still not sure what she's thinking and/or what you did wrong, play back the scenario in your mind and pick it apart, comment by comment, action by action, to look for anything you may have said or done to solicit her anger.

Essential

If you really can't figure it out, run it by a trusting (and honest) friend who doesn't have ADHD. He doesn't have to be a guru or a mind reader, just someone with average sensitivity. He'll probably be able to tell you what you did or said to make your wife react the way she did.

Remember that if something you or your spouse said or did strikes you as inconsistent with your normal or typical reactions or interactions, you're probably getting warmer and closer to isolating the offending comment or behavior.

If You're Stumped, Just Ask

If you can't figure out what you did or said to hurt your wife, you need to ask her to explain. Tell her you need her to explain it in words, and not to respond by sending you more nonverbal cues you won't be able to translate.

Be sure you let her know you welcome her feedback, or she may be reluctant to offer it again. Instead of being defensive or argumentative, listen carefully to what she has to say, incorporate any lessons you've learned, and try to think of it as an opportunity to learn new skills. Don't blame yourself for not being able to read her nonverbal clues.

If, despite these techniques, you still have problems reading nonverbal cues, consult your therapist about other tools and resources that can help you become a better nonverbal translator.

Slowing a Racing Mind

Along with wandering minds, many ADHD adults have racing thoughts that make it difficult to focus, pay attention, be selective, relax, and fall asleep. Unfortunately, stimulant medications—the most common treatment for adult ADHD—often exacerbate the problem. Clonidine, an antihypertensive agent, is often prescribed in adult ADHD cases to be taken late in the day. It is believed to help with both ADHD symptoms and with relaxation and sleep.

Natural Calming Agents

From exercise to Eastern medicine, there are many ways to rein in runaway thoughts. Aerobic exercise can help slow racing thoughts by releasing endorphins, hormones that enhance feelings of well-being and calm. Exercise also helps you shake off the anxiety, stress, and fear that can trigger racing thoughts.

Meditation, deep breathing, yoga, and tai chi slow runaway thoughts by teaching you to focus on the natural internal rhythms of inhaling and exhaling. Learning to keep your thoughts in the "now" can reduce anxiety and stress, both of which trigger worrying, fretting, and racing thoughts about the unknown. Calming music can also help slow down racing thoughts and help you keep your thoughts in the present.

Fact

Exercise that entails a high degree of presence, focus, concentration, and hand-eye coordination, such as rock climbing and kayaking, can help slow racing thoughts by literally crowding them out of your brain. Extremely rigorous sports like marathon running or cycling can also alleviate racing thoughts by forcing you to stay focused on the present situation and by releasing endorphins.

Enjoyable mental escapes that capture your attention can also help shift your focus away from worrying, racing thoughts and toward your escape of choice. Mental escapes can range from cooking and crossword puzzles to video games and movies.

Making Friends

Unfortunately, adults with ADHD may find that making and keeping friends takes a great deal of energy and focus. Afraid they'll do the wrong thing, butt in when they're not wanted, or misread nonverbal cues and make a serious social faux pas, ADHD adults often find socializing to be more draining than rewarding and relaxing.

ADHD-Friendly Ways to Make and Keep Friends

Everyone needs friends, especially ADHD adults. If your symptoms have made it difficult or challenging for you to make meaningful friendships and maintain them during troubled times, you may be going about it in the wrong way. Here are some strategies to help you make and keep friendships that can sustain you through good times and bad.

❑ Pick your activities carefully and avoid those that stress or wear you out. Instead, choose those you enjoy the most and find most relaxing. You're already working hard enough to pay attention, focus, concentrate, and read nonverbal cues without forcing yourself to do something you dislike. Engaging in an activity you don't enjoy will only cause you to get bored and tune out or drift away.

❏ Give your brain a rest. Avoid social gatherings or activities that are likely to stress you out because they require maintaining strict focus during lengthy and/or complex conversations. This can include large dinner parties where you're expected to participate in conversation, long lectures that cover complex or unfamiliar material, or foreign movies or operas with subtitles that compel you to follow a plot being spoken or sung in a foreign language. Better bets for ADHD adults include social activities like movies, concerts, and dramatic productions that revolve around passively listening and watching rather than actively participating.

❏ Go for the sports. Attending a sporting event gives you the opportunity to get up, move around, or go grab a hot dog and soda without disturbing the other spectators. Participating in sports lets you blow off stress and anxiety.

❏ Choose "active" dining activities. Rather than formal sit-down dinners that may revolve around long conversations, choose more informal dining engagements, such as buffets, outdoor barbecue and pool parties, potluck parties, or casual dinners centered around home or rental movies. These options offer more chances for hyperactive types to get up and move around and for inattentive types to focus on short, informal conversations with people of their choosing.

❏ Practice being a pal. Making and keeping friends requires time and effort on your part, so don't expect friendships to flourish in a vacuum. Make staying in touch with friends easy and fast by creating a master list of names, phone numbers, and e-mails on your computer. Set aside some time every week to touch base with close friends and set up lunch dates or activities with those who live nearby. If you have limited time for staying in touch, remember that it's better to make a quick phone call or send a short e-mail than to do nothing at all.

❑ Surprise your friends on important dates. Your thoughtfulness in remembering birthdays, anniversaries, and special occasions will go a long way toward cementing relationships. To keep track of dates and send gifts with the touch of a button, use an online service like *www.birthdayalarm .com*.

❑ Flex your creative muscles. If you're artistic, make your own cards. They're practically guaranteed to win a place of honor on the recipients' refrigerator or mirror. Use your creativity to make unusual, one-of-a-kind gifts, such as homemade cookies and fudge. Or use your imagination to buy something for a friend you know she would never buy for herself, such as a beautiful vase, a massage at a local day spa, a signed first edition hardcover written by her favorite author, or a gift coupon for dinner at a gourmet restaurant.

Should I Tell My Friends I Have ADHD?

Many ADHD adults struggle with whether to tell friends they have the disorder. Some believe it is better that friends understand what they are going through so they can be more understanding and flexible when their symptoms flare up. Others worry that telling friends they have adult ADHD will scare them away or cause friends to start treating them with kid gloves.

According to experts, there's really no one right answer. In many cases, the right decision may be based on the severity of your symptoms, and/or the closeness of the relationship.

When Your Symptoms Are Mild

If your symptoms are mild and you are able to manage or disguise most of them with medication and therapy, you may decide there's no reason to tell friends you have adult ADHD unless you feel that telling them would strengthen your friendship.

When Your Symptoms Are Severe

On the other hand, if your symptoms are more severe and/or frequently disrupt your life and the lives of others, telling friends you have the condition may help them be more understanding, forgiving, and flexible when they're on the receiving end of your symptoms.

Telling a Prospective Spouse

It's always wise to reveal your disorder when you're dating someone who is highly likely to become a permanent life partner. Adult ADHD can negatively impact everything from your ability to earn a living or regulate your moods to your capacity for intimacy. The disorder is also hereditary.

If you're contemplating marriage with someone you're dating, telling him about your adult ADHD and coming up with a plan for how the two of you can deal with it before any issues arise can strengthen your relationship. Be honest with him about how your symptoms may impact your marriage, your capacity to get and keep a meaningful and well-paying job, your ability to be comfortable during intimacy, and how being an ADHD parent will affect your potential children (who are at a high risk of inheriting the disorder).

CHAPTER 17

Harmony on the Home Front

Without professional intervention, adult ADHD can turn even the happiest home into a never-ending battlefront. Adult ADHD's core symptoms of disorganization, distraction, inattention, and impulsivity can unravel the fabric of family life and cause emotional, mental, physical, and financial turmoil for everyone involved. Children of ADHD parents are at an increased risk of growing up in broken homes, and the spouses of adults with ADHD are often stretched to the breaking point.

An Hour in the Life of an ADHD Parent or Spouse

If you're an ADHD adult, you already know that even the smallest household chores can require a lot more time and effort for you to accomplish than your non-ADHD spouse. If you're not, you may have no idea what a mere hour in the life of someone struggling with this disorder may look like.

An Adult ADHD Chain of Events

Let's say your wife calls you at work and tells you that she's run out of a few essential ingredients to finish making dinner, and wonders if you could pick them up on your way home. For a non-ADHD spouse, this would be a simple matter of stopping by the supermarket, picking up the items, and delivering them to his wife.

But as an ADHD adult, you have several hurdles to clear before you even get out the door of your office. First, if you're particularly interested in what you're doing at work, you have to break your hyperfocus, tell yourself that you can pick up where you left off tomorrow, and leave yourself some sort of note or clue as to where to begin working.

Because you're so disorganized, it may take you some time to figure out how to make sure you won't lose all the work you've already done before leaving for the day. Faced with that task, you may hyperfocus on that and spend so much time making sure you'll be able to find your place tomorrow that you lose all track of time and wind up starting out for the grocery store too late. If you make it to the grocery store on time, you may forget what your wife wanted you to buy because you didn't write it down.

Instead of calling her back, you may have impulsively decided to try to remember the items she wanted by walking up and down the aisles until something jogged your memory, spending an hour wandering the aisles for what should have taken you five minutes. By the time you get home with the items, you're exhausted and frazzled from the search, your wife is angry and disappointed that you couldn't buy a few simple things, and your children are irritable, disgruntled, tired, and maybe still hungry.

Essential

Writing things down tends to go against the natural instinct of most people with ADHD because it entails paying attention. Memory experts agree, though, that the more senses you use to store something in your memory, the better you'll be able to recall it later. Write a list to increase your odds of remembering it.

After dinner, because neither you nor your wife has the energy to help the kids with their homework, they plant themselves in front of the television set and fall asleep before cracking their textbooks. The next day, the teacher calls you and wants to know why your children never complete their homework.

Adult ADHD Intervention Tactics

Regardless of how adult ADHD has unraveled your family or marriage in the past, it's possible to do damage control and get things in order by having everyone in the family master some basic coping techniques and skills.

Try a Little Tenderness

Family members can gain valuable insight from putting themselves in the ADHD adult's place. Until everyone in the family understands that their ADHD spouse or parent isn't intentionally screwing up, forgetting to show up, failing to pay attention, or neglecting to listen, they will assume that he is doing it on purpose.

Fact

Once family members understand that their ADHD spouse or parent is a prisoner of his own symptoms, they can start taking steps to help him minimize his ADHD symptoms and maximize his ADHD strengths.

Family members can also learn how to deal with the volatile emotions, moodiness, bluntness, critical nature, and high frustration levels exhibited by ADHD adults. They need to program themselves not to take things personally and remember that these symptoms are part of the disorder.

Acknowledge and Release Pent-up Feelings

Agree to acknowledge and share how unpredictable symptoms and emotions make you feel rather than bottling them up and letting them fester. In the supermarket scenario, the wife could acknowledge her ADHD husband's shortcomings, including his own frustration at not being able to buy the groceries on time, and help him devise a strategy that can help him master the task next time. Maybe she could make sure he writes down the grocery items, help him develop a way to "flag" his work so he can easily pick up where he left off the next day, call him to remind him it's time to leave for the grocery store, and thank him for the extra effort and coordination it required on his part to pick up the grocery items. This is much more productive than bottling up her increasing frustration with her ADHD husband's inability to do simple chores.

Fact

All non-ADHD family members should recognize their ADHD spouse or parent is operating with some basic mental and emotional deficiencies that make doing simple things very difficult. By having compassion for him and adjusting their expectations and demands so he can succeed, everyone wins.

Give Up the Guilt and Embarrassment

Maybe you feel embarrassed because your ADHD parent forgot to come to your parent-teacher night or insulted your soccer coach for making you sit on the bench. Or perhaps you're embarrassed that your ADHD spouse blurted out something confidential and potentially embarrassing at the block party. Or perhaps you're the ADHD adult and you feel guilty and embarrassed for stepping out of line. It's important for the entire family to recognize that if anything is to blame, it's ADHD itself.

Instead of trying to blame a phantom, family members should help the ADHD parent or spouse mend his ways by helping him get more organized. You could create family calendars, schedules, or timetables, stay more focused on conversations, and rein in impulsive behavior and comments by counting to ten before saying something potentially insulting or embarrassing.

Fact

One way to keep an ADHD spouse or parent organized is to display prominent schedules and timetables at strategic locations throughout the house. Rather than hiding schedules in computer files that are only obvious when opened, post duplicate schedules in the kitchen, in the bedroom, on bathroom mirrors—wherever family members will see them repeatedly and be likely to remember them.

Family members can also help reduce the clutter and disorganization that seems to afflict ADHD adults by designating special places for key items like car keys, credit cards, and garage door openers.

Clearing the Air

ADHD adults are already communication-challenged, for several reasons. Because of their inattention, they have trouble focusing and paying attention, they have poor memories and forget what's already been said, they become bored easily and tune out of conversations they find irrelevant, and they are easily distracted by extraneous noises, music, and uncomfortable physical factors. In addition, their impulsivity and hyperactivity tends to make them speak without thinking first, to blurt out overly blunt statements that hurt or offend others, to butt into conversations without being invited, and to pontificate on topics without realizing everyone else has heard enough.

To prevent communication snafus from coming between family members, it's important that everyone in the family understands the limitations imposed by adult ADHD and finds ways to overcome the communication gaps.

Some snafus can be nipped in the bud by asking for clarification if you don't understand what someone else is asking or requesting. Others can be avoided by acknowledging and repeating what another person has said to make sure you heard and interpreted it correctly. Finally, resist the temptation to criticize, which tends to reduce or shut down communication by building walls or creating conflicts that disguise the real issue at hand.

If there's a chance a distracted ADHD spouse or parent may forget an important meeting, have everyone in the family synchronize the alarms on their watches or cell phones so they all buzz at once. Then everyone can call, text, or e-mail Mom or Dad.

Practicing Thanks and Gratitude

Everyone needs to be appreciated, acknowledged, and thanked for their accomplishments, achievements, and attempts, especially ADHD adults who are so accustomed to being criticized that they are hard-wired for blame, accusations, and negativity and are understandably defensive, withdrawn, and unable to express affection.

Essential

To create lasting family bonds, encourage family members to express love, appreciation, thanks, and support on a daily basis to the ADHD adult through hugs, smiles, pats on the back, a thumbs up, kind words, and simple thanks.

It's also amazing what a little humor can do to defuse a potentially embarrassing or difficult situation. Instead of focusing on the negative ("You forgot to pay the electric bill and now we're all going to freeze to death tonight!") lighten up and reframe it as a funny episode that will go down in time in the family scrapbook. ("No heat tonight, so let's use it as an excuse to have a fun family night out at the local motel, where they keep the thermostat so high we'll probably have to open all the windows!")

Alleviating Conflicts and Disruption

Ask anyone who has ADHD or lives with someone who does and you'll probably get the same response: At times, it can seem like adult ADHD is synonymous with conflict and disruption. The disorder often creates nonstop chaos and havoc in practically every area and aspect of the home, turning what should be a relaxing escape for family members into a never-ending battlefield.

The Star in Her Own Soap Opera

One reason so many adults with ADHD are routinely mired in conflict is that one symptom of the disorder is a compulsion to create chaos as a substitute for excitement and drama.

Fact

In their attempts to stir up the dust so they remain the center of attention, ADHD adults often fabricate problems and dramas that are not one-act plays but rather convoluted, long-running soap operas that repeat themselves over and over again as problems and issues change size or shape but never seem to reach any real resolution.

Families can pull the plug on ADHD-inspired soap operas by sitting down with a family therapist and getting to the bottom of why the ADHD adult feels compelled to spin out soap operas. Once the sufferer and her family members understand the emotional voids the dramas are intended to fill, they can help boost her self-esteem, increase her confidence, and replace her energy-draining dramas with more productive activities that can strengthen, rather than deflate, her resources.

Understanding and Recognizing the Root of Mood Swings

In addition to her constant need for drama, an ADHD adult is also likely to suffer from periodic or chronic mood swings. It's important for family members to understand that these mood swings are often not connected to or triggered by a particular event or person, but may be the result of neurobiological imbalances, waxing and waning medication levels, side effects of medications, dietary triggers, and coexisting depression, anxiety, or bipolar disorder.

Essential

ADHD adults are often extremely sensitive to criticism and may put up a wall to protect them from what may feel like a never-ending barrage of criticism. Having disappointed many people over the years and been told countless times they are unpredictable, unreliable, or unproductive, they may react to similar complaints from family members by withdrawing or lashing back.

Many ADHD adults exhaust themselves trying to cope with a never-ending daily parade of symptoms, which can also make them feel helpless, scared, and hopeless.

A family therapist can work with family members and the ADHD adult to take a closer look at mood swings, help isolate likely triggers, eliminate possible causes of these mood swings, and educate the family about mood triggers that may not always be treatable.

Letting Go of the Past

Many ADHD adults live with perpetual feelings of guilt and shame about failures in the past, even if their failures were triggered by undiagnosed ADHD symptoms and not caused by a lack of motivation, laziness, or disinterest. Like a broken record, the song of "failure" replays itself over and over again and often drowns out present-day successes and accomplishments.

By working with a family therapist, family members can help the ADHD adult understand that, until she stops dwelling on past failures and begins to live in the present, she will never be able to replace her gloom-and-doom with feelings of contentment and happiness. Once she realizes it's impossible to undo the past and that the more she is keeping negative thoughts alive by dwelling on them, an ADHD adult can bury the past and open her eyes to the many possibilities, opportunities, and avenues for joy that exist in the present.

Importance of Family Therapy

Adult ADHD is a family problem as well as an individual problem. Because the symptoms of the disorder often wreak havoc on every member of the family, not just the individual with adult ADHD, it's important for the entire group to undergo family therapy, even if the ADHD parent is already getting individual counseling.

Although many families with adult ADHD don't start therapy until a crisis that requires professional intervention occurs, it's best to begin family therapy as soon as it becomes clear that the symptoms of adult ADHD are interfering with normal family functioning. Family therapy can help avoid crises and emergencies that may take months or years to resolve.

Types of Family Therapy

Like individual therapy, there are many different types and styles of family therapy, including therapy that focuses on teaching family members new skills and coping strategies, and therapy in which family members support and encourage each other and learn to communicate more effectively. Many ADHD families participate in ongoing therapy where family members can cycle in and out as necessary to discuss specific needs and challenges. Since adult and childhood ADHD may be present in one family, ADHD families are advised to find a therapist with extensive training, experience, and expertise in adult as well as childhood ADHD.

Finding a Family Therapist

To find a good family therapist, contact a local ADHD support group for referrals, ask your family physician or medical experts for recommendations, or contact local branches of Children and Adults with Attention Deficit/Hyperactivity Disorder (CHADD; *www.chadd.org*). You may also want to ask your insurance provider for a list of therapists in your area who are covered under your plan. Be advised that your insurance company may only cover a set number of visits per year.

CHAPTER 18

Can This Relationship Be Saved?

Marriages in which one or both partners have adult ADHD are twice as likely to end in divorce as other marriages, according to research published in the *Journal of Clinical Psychiatry*. The primary symptoms of adult ADHD can make it difficult for an ADHD spouse to get and keep a job, focus on household tasks like bookkeeping and budgeting, and contribute in a meaningful way to raising and disciplining children. Because ADHD adults crave novelty and excitement, they may have problems remaining faithful to their partner and developing sexual intimacy.

When You or Your Partner Has Adult ADHD

Maintaining a happy and fulfilling marriage is challenging enough without adult ADHD in the mix. But when one or both partners have the disorder, they may lack many of the personal attributes necessary to build a happy and rewarding relationship.

The Cycle of Adult ADHD Marriage

Many ADHD marriages follow a typical cycle that often leads to divorce. The cycle usually begins with the non-ADHD spouse withdrawing from the marriage or relationship because she can no longer cope with the ADHD partner's chronic disorganization, forgetfulness, messiness, clutter, emotional outbursts, and unpredictable or embarrassing behavior or comments. Instead of attempting to help the ADHD spouse, out of sheer exhaustion, frustration, or resentment, she gradually retreats into her job, hobbies, or friends, or she may use an extramarital affair as an escape.

Sensing failure, defeat, or criticism, the ADHD spouse withdraws in turn, and may "hide" or seek relief in extramarital affairs or risky behavior such as substance abuse, alcohol abuse, or gambling. He, too, may seek refuge in his work and hyperfocus on it to the exclusion of everything else, including the needs of the children.

Alert

Many of the spouses of adults with ADHD are trapped in a vicious cycle of anger, resentment, fear, denial, escape, and disappointment that escalates and often leads to separation, divorce, domestic abuse, abandonment of children, and other problems. Without professional help, many couples with an ADHD spouse are doomed to failure.

The non-ADHD spouse responds by becoming angry, suspicious, resentful, disappointed, or disgruntled, and by demanding that the ADHD spouse "clean up his act." This causes the ADHD spouse to become even more aloof, withdrawn, forgetful, distracted, and disorganized, bringing the destructive cycle full circle.

Common Problems in ADHD Marriages

From arguments over money to problems with intimacy and sexuality, there are some common themes in marriages where one or both partners have adult ADHD.

- Many ADHD adults are impulsive spenders who rack up huge credit card debts that threaten the family's financial stability and make saving or planning for long-term goals virtually impossible.

- Many adult ADHD adults have chronic problems at work and are routinely demoted or dismissed because of their inability to concentrate at work, finish projects, work well with others, or accept criticism from superiors. Because ADHD adults are fired far more frequently than non-ADHD adults, they may not earn enough to support a family or contribute to the household.

- Many ADHD adults engage routinely in addictive behavior like drinking, substance abuse, and gambling—habits that can quickly deplete a family's finances and land the ADHD spouse behind bars.

- Because of their impulsive nature and addiction to novelty and thrill-seeking, ADHD spouses are far more likely than other spouses to engage in extramarital affairs. These affairs often threaten the marriage and result in violent arguments, domestic abuse, separation, divorce, and heated child custody suits. Because so many ADHD marriages end in divorce, many children of ADHD marriages end up in broken homes and wind up fending for themselves.

- ADHD spouses often have problems with intimacy for many reasons: an inability to focus or concentrate for long periods of time, hypersensitivity to touch and sound, a tendency to be overly blunt, poor self-esteem, and overuse of alcohol and drugs, which may dull or diminish sexual desire and performance.

- Chronic disorganization and forgetfulness may render an ADHD spouse unreliable and unpredictable when it comes to handling household chores, taking care of and disciplining children, or managing family finances. The non-ADHD spouse is often forced to pick up the slack. She may become very angry and resentful toward her ADHD spouse, or come to view him as another child.

- ADHD spouses tend to leave clutter and messiness in their wake. This can annoy and frustrate spouses and family members and make it difficult for everyone to keep track of things, get and stay organized, and keep the house tidy and clean.
- ADHD spouses often are so distracted and preoccupied by their own thoughts, interests, projects, or problems that they come across as self-centered, selfish, narcissistic, egotistical, or living in a world of their own. Spouses and children may feel overlooked, unappreciated, ignored, dismissed, or unloved. Spouses may look for love and affection outside the marriage, or ask for a separation or divorce.

Understanding Your Partner's Disorder

If you're married to someone who exhibits many adult ADHD symptoms but who has not yet been diagnosed and treated, the first step is to see a professional together.

Once a diagnosis is made, the next task for the non-ADHD spouse is to learn everything she can about the disorder so she understands the symptoms and how her spouse may be as manifesting them at home, at work, and in social settings. The more you know, the more you and any children can better understand your ADHD spouse.

Once you and your spouse and children understand that you're dealing with a disorder rather than character flaws, you should set aside some time to discuss how and why the symptoms have affected your relationship, what each of you can do to stop the vicious cycle from repeating itself, and what type of professional therapy will best help get your marriage back on track.

Steps to Clearing the Air

Honesty is the best policy when it comes to discussing and dealing with a spouse's ADHD symptoms. While there are some things you may have to learn to accept and live with, such as an

ADHD spouse's tendency toward messiness and clutter, it's important to get key grievances and concerns on the table so you can begin addressing them. Here are some steps that may help get the ball rolling in the right direction.

1. Write down a list of grievances, complaints, and things that bother you about each other so you have a permanent record you can refer to and modify as needed. The list of complaints should be a two-way street, not just a litany of criticisms directed at the ADHD partner.

2. Sit down together and make a list of things you want to change about your marriage, including sexual intimacy, communication, and physical improvements such as organizing the household finances or clearing the house of needless clutter. The list could also include suggestions on ways to delegate or break down household chores and tasks so each spouse is responsible for tasks they do best.

3. Keep the tone neutral, not accusatory. Your ADHD spouse has probably suffered from years of blame and criticism and may not be emotionally capable of absorbing more criticism without shutting down or tuning you out. Instead of finger-pointing or blaming, direct your complaints toward the problem, not toward your spouse. For instance, instead of saying "You're such a slob that I can't find anything," you might want to say, "This clutter is making it hard to find anything. Let's figure out a way to get organized so we can find things easier and faster."

4. ADHD adults are masters at creative thinking. Encourage your ADHD spouse to brainstorm ways to tackle problems using creative problem solving.

5. Timing is essential. Schedule constructive conversations for a time of day when your ADHD spouse is most likely to be relaxed and receptive to your suggestions or comments—for instance, after he works out or has had a

chance to unwind from work, rather than right after he gets home.

6. Tackle one problem at a time. Your ADHD spouse may be easily overwhelmed by too many details and may tune out when he has difficulty following your train of thought or when he's listening to a particularly long and complicated discussion or lecture. To make sure your suggestions get through, keep things simple and use short, direct sentences rather than long, convoluted ones. Make sure the topic is of interest to him. If he's extremely interested, his ability to hyperfocus for long periods of time can help you reach a more effective conclusion more quickly.

7. Don't make adult ADHD an excuse for bad behavior. Both partners should recognize and appreciate that, while some adult ADHD symptoms may be annoying, frustrating, and sometimes involuntary, they are not an excuse for bad behavior or inappropriate comments. Also, both people should agree that having the disorder does not give the ADHD spouse license to continue repeating behaviors that are destructive to the marriage simply because they are ADHD symptoms.

8. Be patient with your ADHD spouse and give him the time and support he needs to make necessary changes in his behavior, habits, and thoughts. A combination of medication, therapy, and behavioral modification is often very successful in alleviating symptoms, but don't expect all of his ADHD symptoms to vanish overnight or even altogether.

9. Anticipate temporary setbacks. While the right medication can often bring fast or even immediate improvements in mood, attention, and impulsivity, be prepared to weather some temporary setbacks. Your ADHD spouse and his physician can work together to make necessary adjustments in medication dosage and scheduling to ensure there's always a steady stream of the drug in his bloodstream.

Get It Out in the Open

In a study conducted by Wayne State University on couples where one partner had adult ADHD, non-ADHD spouses said they were most bothered by their spouse's failure to remember what they were told, tendency to zone out on conversations, and inability to take a project from concept to reality. Getting things out in the open can help establish the honest and open communication that is needed to iron out problems and challenges.

When Inattention Invades Relationships

The core symptoms of adult ADHD—inattention, impulsivity, hyperactivity, and disorganization—can manifest in a wide variety of challenging behavior patterns, thinking patterns, and communication problems. Any or all of these symptoms can come between marital partners or lovers who are trying to communicate, get along, or make love. It may sometimes seem as if there's a third person in the room.

Reining in Inattention

Because most ADHD adults are easily bored by things they don't find fascinating or relevant, everyday tasks such as taking out the garbage or changing the light bulbs may remain undone.

Inattentiveness may also manifest as being unable to focus on paying bills on time, being unable to read unspoken cues, or failing to notice when something is wrong. At times, they may come across as self-centered, self-absorbed, and disinterested in everything but themselves. Here are some strategies couples can use by mutual agreement to help an ADHD partner stay focused.

❑ Help the ADHD spouse or partner stay focused by assigning him household chores and tasks he enjoys and does easily.
❑ Keep your spouse organized and on time by writing down important tasks and chores on Post-It notes, bulletin boards,

or elsewhere so he sees the same message several times in the house.

❏ If inattention makes it difficult for your spouse to stay focused during lovemaking, remove anything distracting from the area, whether it's extraneous noise like overly loud music or TV or distracting scents like overly strong perfume. Remember that what might seem exciting or arousing to a non-ADHD spouse can easily distract someone with adult ADHD because of their hypersensitivity to sights, smells, sounds, textures, and touches.

❏ Keep things interesting in your relationship. ADHD adults thrive on variety and newness and tend to wander (emotionally and mentally) when things get boring. To keep things from getting stale in the bedroom, experiment with different positions or try a different room. A little variety will go a long way toward spicing up a relationship.

When Impulsivity Comes Calling

Impulsivity, another common adult ADHD trait, can sometimes make a non-ADHD spouse or lover wonder if he's living with or married to a five-year-old child. Impulsive ADHD spouses and partners often have little patience for things that don't go their way and are likely to lose their cool or blow their temper during difficult or challenging times.

Putting a Lid on Impulsivity

Because ADHD adults are drawn to excitement and novelty, their impulsivity can manifest as risky, thrill-seeking impulsive behavior. Impulsive spending, gambling, driving, drinking or drug use, and illicit sex are just a few impulsive activities that can unravel a relationship.

The following are some strategies for dealing with impulsive behavior in ADHD partners.

❏ Keep your cool and avoid escalating arguments. Because adult ADHD spouses thrive on drama, they may actually enjoy arguing for the sake of it and may unconsciously look for ways to prolong an argument until it provokes dramatic emotions.

❏ Help prevent embarrassing behavior in social settings by acting as your partner's eyes and ears. Work out a series of unobtrusive signals between the two of you—like raising an eyebrow or stroking your chin—so you can warn your ADHD spouse ahead of time that he's on thin ice.

❏ Introduce "safe" impulsive behavior into your relationship to take the place of dangerous impulsivity. If your partner craves excitement, look for exciting, thrill-seeking activities you can do together, such as white-water rafting, bungee jumping, downhill skiing, or cycling.

When Hyperactivity Runs You Ragged

Hyperactivity can manifest itself as extreme restlessness, an inability to sit still, racing thoughts, and chronic fidgeting and squirming. Hyperactivity can make it difficult for ADHD partners to pay attention, stay focused, follow and track lengthy conversations, do one thing for any lengthy of time, and quiet their minds so they can relax and enjoy activities that require lingering or hanging out.

Preventing Hyperactivity from Wreaking Havoc

One way to prevent hyperactivity from running your relationship ragged is to make sure your ADHD partner takes his medications in a proper and timely fashion. Many ADHD medications slow racing minds and produce feelings of calm and tranquility.

The following are some other nonmedical strategies that may help calm hyperactivity in your ADHD significant other.

❏ Avoid activities that force your ADHD partner to sit perfectly still and quiet for long periods of time, such as going to the cinema, attending theater or opera performances, or going to formal dinners.

❑ Enjoy activities that allow your ADHD partner to get up, move around, and stretch his legs frequently. This may include athletic events like baseball or football games where it's easy to stand up to cheer, buy a hot dog, or use the restroom. Active sports like cycling and hiking are also ideal in that they let your partner move around, limit the amount of socializing he has to do, and burn off nervous energy. As a side bonus, exercise also releases calming, feel-good endorphins.

❑ Help your ADHD partner slow his racing mind and stay in the present by encouraging him to take up yoga, tai chi, deep breathing exercise, and/or walking meditation. Even better, do these activities together.

When Disorganization Divides Couples

ADHD partners often suffer from chronic disorganization. External clutter is often a tip-off that their brains are cluttered and disorganized as well.

Disorganized Thinking

ADHD disorganization usually extends to the way ADHD partners think and function. It may include an inability to organize, prioritize, or plan ahead; having no sense of time or deadlines; and an inability to divide complex tasks into several smaller steps.

The following are some strategies that can help put a lid on disorganization.

❑ Help your partner de-clutter by tackling one room at a time (or one corner of one room at a time if things are really bad) and clearing the decks of anything he doesn't need or use. Organize a yard or garage sale and make a profit on his excesses.

❏ Create holding tanks for everyday household items that are likely to get scattered and lost throughout the house. Put a basket by the door for sunglasses, wallets, or briefcases and hang a hook by the door for house and car keys. Make sure your ADHD partner places these items in the proper place the minute he walks into the house.

❏ Put it in writing. Create a master chart for the week that includes all tasks, chores, appointments, meetings, doctor's appointments, etc. It can also be an easy reference for important phone numbers, e-mails, and other contact information.

How to Keep Romance Alive

While sexual desire is certainly an important ingredient in romantic life, without trust, respect, understanding, and empathy between partners, romance and sexual desire can wither and die.

When Trust Dies, the Marriage Often Follows

Many ADHD relationships fall apart when an ADHD partner betrays her partner's trust by lying and cheating to fulfill a craving for novelty and excitement. If you and your partner are caught in a cycle of distrust, consider working with a therapist to reestablish healthy boundaries for your relationship, discussing what triggered the betrayal, figuring out strategies to keep it from happening again, and learning to forgive and forget.

I Don't Get No Respect

Many ADHD adults are extremely sensitive to criticism and blame. Belittling, degrading, or continually criticizing an ADHD partner is guaranteed to demolish a romance, especially if the ADHD partner is struggling to overcome the very ADHD symptoms you are criticizing.

When ADHD is a third party in a relationship, both partners can prevent criticism and blame from overriding romance by supporting the ADHD partner and building up self-esteem and self-confidence.

Listen and Focus on the Positive

When you're married to a person with a disorder as complicated and potentially destructive as ADHD, it can be easy to see the many things that are wrong with the relationship and become negative, bitter, or discouraged. In addition, many ADHD adults also struggle with depression, low self-esteem, and a lack of confidence. Their pessimism can wear down the spirits of even the sunniest spouse.

 Alert

Negativity has a nasty habit of feeding on itself. The more you look for negatives, the more negatives you see and the more negative things tend to become. Also, focusing on negatives doesn't leave any time or energy for focusing on the positive. To break the destructive cycle, make a concerted effort to look at the bright side.

To prevent negativity from sinking your relationship, focus on your partner's many positive ADHD attributes. For instance, perhaps she's creative, spontaneous, or always eager to try something new, while you tend to be overly conservative and cautious. Look at the many ways she enriches and enlivens your life. Once you shift your attitude, don't be surprised to see an increase in her positive feelings and behaviors.

Acknowledge and Resolve Conflicts

Raging thoughts and impulsivity make it difficult for many ADHD adults not to jump to conclusions or restrain themselves from interrupting a conversation before their partner has a chance to speak her mind, explain, or clarify.

Essential

You may become frustrated when you don't understand or can't follow your partner's thoughts. Instead of focusing on what you thought she said, ask her to repeat or clarify her statement so there's no second-guessing and confusion on your part.

If you disagree with something your spouse has said, speak your mind rather than giving in for the sake of avoiding an argument. If you always give in, you'll eventually erode your sense of self and feel as if you've given up your voice and power, which can leave you resenting your spouse.

Walk a Mile in Your Partner's Shoes

Empathy is the ability to understand how it feels to be in someone else's situation. If your spouse has ADHD, empathize with the many challenges and struggles she copes with on a daily basis and try to understand things from her perspective.

If you're unable to put yourself in your spouse's shoes, you may build a wall between you that blocks out honesty and openness. A marriage counselor can help you and your spouse examine and break down the barriers that are interfering with communication and intimacy.

How Adult ADHD Affects Sexual Intimacy

When ADHD enters the bedroom, distraction, wandering thoughts, and a lack of desire usually aren't far behind. In fact, sexual boredom is one of the biggest complaints among ADHD couples, and a major reason behind their high divorce rate. Unfortunately, even when couples are sexually active, ADHD symptoms can interfere with emotional and sexual intimacy, leaving one or both partners feeling unconnected, alone, and sexually frustrated or unsatisfied.

When ADHD and Sex Don't Mix

Hurt feelings, confusion, and resentment can build and fester when one or both partners feel emotionally and/or sexually unsatisfied. If misinformation or misunderstanding is the main culprit, a marriage counselor or sex therapist can help the non-ADHD spouse understand how the disorder affects sexual desire and performance.

Essential

Sly Stone wasn't kidding when he sang about "different strokes for different folks," even if he wasn't talking about ADHD partners. The fact is, what may feel pleasurable to a non-ADHD spouse may be downright irritating, annoying, or even painful to an ADHD partner who is hypersensitive to the touches, tastes, smells, and sounds that come into play during sex.

For instance, many ADHD partners are too hyperactive to relax and get in the mood. Instead of shutting out the world and focusing on their partner, they're distracted by their racing thoughts. Others are distracted by loud music, even if it's romantic. Instead of focusing on their partner, they may start singing along or talking about how much they loved the last concert.

How to Improve Sexual Intimacy

Provided there aren't emotional distractions or barriers interfering with intimacy, it's possible to overcome distractions that may prevent an ADHD spouse from being able to focus on, respond to, or enjoy sexual intimacy.

The following are some strategies for turning up the heat in your ADHD marriage or relationship.

- Talk openly about what turns your ADHD spouse on—and off. If she's super-sensitive to scented oils or lotions, finds music more distracting than romantic, or can't stand your scratchy beard, get rid of it.
- Be open to new experiences. ADHD adults love novelty, so don't be afraid to introduce something new to ward off ADHD boredom. Make sure you're both comfortable with it before trying anything. If your ADHD spouse isn't comfortable with it, it's likely to become yet another ADHD distraction.
- Practice being in the moment. To help your hyperactive partner stay in the now, try doing yoga, tai chi, meditation, deep breathing exercises, or massage as a couple. Then move the relaxed togetherness into the bedroom.
- Let go of libido-killers. When ADHD symptoms make your ADHD spouse unreliable, it may force you into assuming the role of parent. Once the child/parent pattern becomes the norm in a relationship, romance and sexuality between partners usually declines. If you and your partner are trapped in this pattern, work with a therapist to rebalance your relationship so you're both equal partners.
- Make a date. If conflicting schedules are preventing you and your partner from having fun together, playing together, or hooking up, make a date and put it on the calendar. Then commit to it.

Lasting Happiness and Love

While ADHD poses disadvantages in a relationship, it also has many advantages. Opposites often attract, so if you're the steady, reliable, and dependable type who could use a jolt of spontaneity, impulsivity, novelty, and excitement, an ADHD spouse may be just what the doctor ordered. On the other hand, if you're an ADHD adult who has trouble balancing his checkbook, matching his socks, or remembering to feed the dog, a non-ADHD spouse could be the gift from heaven you've been searching for.

While it may take some effort, it's possible for an ADHD relationship to have a happy and permanent ending. An ADHD spouse needs to take responsibility for his disorder rather than use it as an excuse for his problems.

In addition, the non-ADHD spouse needs to remember that she's married to someone who's wired a little differently than most people. While an ADHD marriage may not always run like clockwork, it could be a lot more lively and fun.

CHAPTER 19

Overcoming Workplace and Career Challenges

Adult ADHD symptoms can wreak havoc on your job or career. Research shows that many ADHD adults have a spotty work history and are more likely to get demoted or fired than others. Studies also show ADHD adults change jobs far more frequently than non-ADHD adults. Viewed as unreliable, they may end up in low-paying jobs that don't capitalize on their intellectual or creative potential.

Major Workplace Challenges

The workplace presents a variety of special challenges for ADHD adults. Because of their tendency to become distracted, they have trouble focusing on work-related tasks they find boring, dull, or routine, and may neglect or forget to complete them before moving on to something else that is more interesting.

Inattention may make it difficult for them to track conversations or follow instructions. Hyperactivity can make sitting at their desk or through a long meeting practically impossible, and may also cause them to fidget or otherwise disrupt other workers.

Procrastination is another serious problem for ADHD adults, many of whom can't begin working on a project until they have the stress of a deadline. Others may be so overwhelmed by a project that they simply put it off because they don't know where to begin.

Impulsivity may lead ADHD adults to say inappropriate or irrelevant things during meetings or to their colleagues or boss, and it may also cause inappropriate and untimely outbursts of temper.

Alert

ADHD adults work an average of twenty-two days a year less than non-ADHD employees because of chronic problems with concentration, distraction, organization, forgetfulness, and impulsiveness. They average 8.4 sick days per year and 21.7 work days associated with a reduction in work because of ADHD symptoms. According to the World Health Organization, 4 percent of adults worldwide may not realize they have adult ADHD.

Eight Work-Related Problem Areas

Adult ADHD symptoms can disrupt a wide range of executive functions and also cause problems with emotional, intellectual, and even physical functioning at work. Here are eight areas that pose special challenges for ADHD adults.

1. Organization skills, including organizing your desk and work day, organizing specific tasks and skills, prioritizing tasks, and dividing big projects into smaller, doable pieces.
2. Long-range planning, or being able to develop and articulate long-range goals at work. ADHD adults also have trouble planning ahead and following through on large projects with multiple deadlines.
3. Staying the course, or being able to remain focused on what needs doing and follow through on it until it's completed.
4. Finding a good middle ground, or being able to establish a work pace and style that enables you to get things done without hyperfocusing. Many ADHD adults routinely work

overtime because they waited until the last minute to start, or didn't understand instructions and did things wrong the first time.

5. Being able to grasp the big picture or overall goal as well as stay focused on the day-to-day tasks without becoming overwhelmed, restless, or distracted.

6. Staying on an even keel, or managing your emotions, controlling your temper, and taking responsibility for your actions.

7. Working well with colleagues, or being able to listen, compromise, delegate, control your temper, maintain a sense of decorum, and function as a team or solo player depending on the situation.

8. Dealing with authority figures, being able to take advice, handle criticism, and follow instructions from a boss without becoming belligerent, defensive, or losing your temper.

Finding a Compatible Career

Adult ADHD doesn't have to come between you and your preferred profession or vocation.

Reality Checks and Balances

The most important thing to remember if you have adult ADHD is that you can find a career in any field you set your mind on. But it is important for you to do a reality check before deciding to embark on a specific professional track.

For instance, many ADHD adults are notoriously bad at bookkeeping and accounting because they find it excruciatingly boring. If you're among them, you probably won't want to embark on a career that involves adding lots of numbers.

The trick is to figure out if you're the type of person that thrives in a creative, fast-paced, and somewhat unpredictable environment like a news room or film set, or if you'd be happier in a quiet, structured, and predictable setting like a library or a research facility.

Find a Career Counselor

If you're not sure where to start your search, you might consider hiring a career counselor or coach. A psychologist can administer a neuropsychological evaluation that yields insights into your cognitive strengths and weaknesses. This test can help you better understand what type of mind you have. A career coach can give you a battery of fun tests that identify your key interests, likes, dislikes, strengths, and weaknesses.

Don't get frustrated if it takes several weeks or months to land your ideal career. It's better to take your time and be sure rather than plunge into yet another job that's wrong for you and end up unhappy and unfulfilled.

Fact

Being excited about a prospective job is contagious to prospective employers. Even if you don't have the strongest resume, your enthusiasm and excitement alone could land you the job if you go into the interview with an upbeat, can-do attitude.

It may also pay to practice your interview techniques. If, like many ADHD adults, you have low self-esteem, practice telling prospective employers about your strengths as they apply to the job at hand. Tell them what and how you would make valuable contributions, and be sure to tell them how much you love the work.

Avoid Black or White Thinking

If a career has certain components that frighten you, or that you fear may be difficult because of your ADHD symptoms, don't let this stop you. You can always find ways to handle the less-than-exciting, boring, or mundane parts of a job.

The tips and strategies outlined in this book will help you get to meetings on time, develop systemized and organized files, and stay calm and collected in the face of deadlines.

Striking Out on Your Own

If you're an ADHD adult who's had problems dealing with authority figures, interpreting office politics, or knowing when to keep your mouth shut, having your own business may seem like the perfect solution. In fact, the creativity, inventiveness, and hyperfocus that are typical of ADHD adults make them ideal entrepreneurs—and quite a few are also self-made millionaires.

Pros and Cons of Being an Entrepreneur

Being your own boss can eliminate some of the struggles and hassles of working for someone else. It also means you won't have to endure office politics, deal with an unrealistic boss, and spend hours doing things you dislike for the sake of making a living.

However, being a successful entrepreneur requires a number of skills that many ADHD adults find difficult, such as focusing, paying attention, working well with others, being able to delegate, reading nonverbal cues, staying motivated through good times and bad, and, of course, being savvy about finance, budgeting, and accounting.

Before making the leap, you might want to talk to other ADHD adults who have started their own businesses.

Getting a Handle on Executive Functions

For many ADHD adults, the biggest work-related challenge is handling and mastering the wide range of executive functions required of them. This includes organizing, prioritizing, delegating, planning, meeting deadlines, and conceptualizing long-range plans and goals.

Strategies to Improve Executive Functions

Staying focused is probably the biggest executive challenge for ADHD adults. That's because to get anything accomplished, you have to stay focused, concentrate, and stick with it until it's finished. Unfortunately, ADHD adults find it difficult to pay attention, especially when they find the subject boring, dull, repetitive, or uninteresting. Instead of focusing, their mind wanders.

Fact

Many ADHD adults struggle to find a healthy balance at work. Some hyperfocus on their work to the exclusion of everything else and become workaholics, while others can't focus at work and are forced to bring work home. While the second group may appear to be workaholics, they are actually compensating for the hours they spend daydreaming or idle at work.

The end result is that the project or task doesn't get done on time—or at all. ADHD adults have to work late or take work home on weekends to complete it. Others become so distracted that they eventually find they have no job at all to focus on.

Here are some tips and strategies to improve your executive functions.

- Centralize your important information. Use a desk calendar, personal organization system, or computer calendar to keep all your essential dates, appointments, reminders, to-do lists, and deadlines in one central location.
- Buy an easy-to-use filing system with color-coded three-sided folders to organize your important projects into separate tasks. Don't use manila envelopes, as materials may fall out of the sides and get lost in the shuffle.
- Start each day by clearing the decks. De-clutter your desk, file important documents, and clear out and file materials in

your in- and outboxes. If something is urgent, tackle it immediately before you forget about it or get distracted.

- Avoid wasting time. Organize projects or tasks on your day calendar and give each task a specific length of time. Don't underestimate. Choose a few of the most essential tasks, prioritize them, and then tackle one at time. If you tend to forget appointments, set multiple alarms on your wristwatch, computer, or cell phone to remind you.

- Develop a methodical system for big projects. To tackle large or long-term projects, develop a systematic approach. Outline the goal of the project and detail major considerations like interim deadlines. Then break the project down into smaller steps and determine how much time each will take, making sure your estimates are realistic and in line with those short-term deadlines. Tackle one task at a time, and give yourself small rewards when each task is completed. Periodically review your timeline to make sure you have enough time to get the project done on time. If it doesn't seem possible, delegate some tasks to others if you're in a position to do so, or approach your boss about getting an extension.

- Do the things you least want to do first thing in the day, if only for a set amount of time each day. You'll find it satisfying and rewarding to move on to tasks you find more enjoyable.

- Hire an organizing genie. If you have trouble organizing and prioritizing, consider hiring a professional organizer to help. For more information, visit the National Association of Professional Organizers (*www.napo.net*).

- Tune out distractions. If you work in a busy or noisy office, it may be difficult for you to focus. If you're distracted by noise or people talking, talk to your boss about using headsets or a white noise machine. If you tend to gaze out the window, pull the blinds. Use visual reminders to help yourself stay alert and focused on tasks. Shake off tension and stress that may disrupt your focus by taking a breather every hour or so. Stretch your arms and legs, shrug your shoulders, scrunch your neck, wiggle your fingers, take some deep breaths, or do some yoga.

- Create a daily to-do list. To manage the many details of your job, write every one down, no matter how small or insignificant, and put the list somewhere you'll be able to see it. Do one at a time. Draw a line through each task as you complete it. You will feel some satisfaction each time you cross off a line, and you will also see that you are making progress. This reinforcement leads to further progress. Make sure to consult your to-do list throughout the day so you don't get sidetracked.

- Remember that organizational strategies may periodically break down, so don't expect perfection. The good news is that once you've established an organizational technique or experienced an organizational success, it becomes easier to reintroduce it and come up with additional strategies for future projects. Expecting permanent or virtually perfect solutions can lead to frustration, recrimination, and loss of self-esteem. Sometimes it's better to accept a less-than-ideal solution and pat yourself on the back for progress you've made.

Learn to Be on Time

Whether it's being on time for work or getting a project done on time, many ADHD adults struggle with meeting deadlines. One reason is that ADHD adults tend to underestimate how long it actually takes to accomplish something. In addition, their chronic disorganization and clutter prevents them from acting efficiently.

Fact

It's not impossible to break the lateness habit, but it will take some effort and practice on your part. Make a deal with yourself to break bad habits. Don't fall into the trap of thinking you can finish just one more thing before you leave.

Until you break the lateness habit, double or even triple the amount of time you think something will take. To become more realistic about how long certain tasks take, write down time estimates in your calendar, and then compare them to actual times after you complete the task. Reset your estimation on your next project to include the extra time. The more you record and correct how long it takes you to do something, the better you'll become at narrowing the gap between how long you think it will take to accomplish something and how long it actually takes.

Working Well with Peers and Superiors

Adult ADHD symptoms may inhibit your ability to appropriately interact with others at work, be a good team player, handle criticism, deal with authority figures, and conduct yourself appropriately during meetings. These factors often play a significant role in how others perceive you and can be the difference between getting promoted and getting fired.

Managing Your Emotions

Many ADHD adults have fragile egos. If your self-esteem is wobbly, you need to be especially careful about acting defensive, continually putting yourself down, or letting other people's perceptions or opinions of you affect your conduct.

Instead of letting a bad temper or inappropriate comments jeopardize your job and work relations, practice staying in tune with how you really feel. Communicate your thoughts to colleagues when necessary.

Managing the Effects of Low Self-Esteem

Many ADHD adults have low self-esteem, and this can manifest in the workplace in a variety of negative ways that can be detrimental to establishing, maintaining, or advancing your career. For instance, low self-esteem may cause you to be to overly concerned about or sensitive to what others think or feel about you, causing you to put your time and energy into more worrying than working.

Essential

Sometimes, poor self-esteem can actually cause you to lose your job. When you don't trust and believe in yourself, it's difficult for others to believe in you. If you talk and behave in a way that continually tells others you think you're worthless, sooner or later your boss may agree with you.

Your low self-esteem may cause you to be very self-critical, defensive when it comes to accepting criticism, or angry because you feel you aren't valued or appreciated. A therapist can help you uncover some of the reasons or dysfunctional thinking behind your poor self-esteem and help you look for ways to improve or bolster it.

Dealing with Authority Figures

Many ADHD adults have trouble dealing with bosses and superiors. Despite all evidence to the contrary, many ADHD adults simply believe they are right about everything most of the time, and that other people are wrong most of the time. Before you let your stubbornness get the best of you, you may want to consider the possibility that you could actually be wrong this time (or any time).

If you still think you're right and your boss is wrong, think carefully about what confronting your boss would accomplish, taking into consideration his personal track record and your personal relationship with him. Would he be likely to listen and thank you for your input, or even be so impressed by your insight that he'd change his mind? Or would he be more likely to be annoyed and insulted that you had the nerve to defy him?

Discovering Your Work-Related Strengths and Weaknesses

Adult ADHD can hamper your ability to look at yourself realistically and gauge your strengths and weaknesses. Not knowing what you're good at (or bad at) can impact your work performance in many ways.

You may struggle with a job because it doesn't match your innate talents, or become bored, disgruntled, or disappointed when your efforts don't yield the results you had expected. A good therapist can help you zone in on your strengths and weaknesses so you can minimize your shortcomings and maximize your many gifts. In fact, many ADHD adults decide to change careers after working with a therapist and wind up in a different job that better fits their ADHD skills and temperament.

Getting in Sync with Office Politics

Being in touch with office politics, knowing how to translate what your superiors are really saying, and understanding your role in the bigger scheme of things are all important strategies for preserving your job.

Because of their inability to read nonverbal cues, their tendency to blurt out inappropriate comments, and their difficulty in working well with others, many ADHD adults are out of the loop when it comes to office politics.

The fact is that success at work is often a case of who you know, not what you know.

Tips for Getting in the Loop

Here are some strategies that will help keep you in the loop and prevent you from becoming an unwitting victim of office politics.

❑ Ask colleagues to rephrase or otherwise clarify important points. Because you're unable to read between the lines of a conversation, you may misunderstand what is actually being said or done. If you aren't sure you really heard the message, ask someone to rephrase it, repeat it, or clarify it until you're positive you get it.

❑ Develop a network of trusted work allies who can translate for you. Just as you'd want to take someone to a party to interpret body language and small talk, you may want to develop a network of friends at work who can interpret office politics for you—especially if it's going to impact your position.

❑ Even better, it's not as difficult as you might think to learn to read nonverbal cues and body language yourself. You can hire a body language expert to teach you or pick up nuances by reading books or attending seminars on the topic. Practice at home by watching a foreign movie with the English subtitles off and then watch it again with the subtitles on to see what you lost in translation.

Stay Focused at Boring Meetings

It's hard for anyone to weather a long, boring meeting without drifting off. But for an ADHD adult, the threat is even greater because of symptoms of inattention, which makes it difficult to follow long conversations, and hyperactivity, which makes it difficult to sit still for long periods of time.

Essential

Break up long, tedious meetings by escaping to the restroom. Try splashing water on your face to clear your head, swinging your arms to release tension, or doing standing push-ups against a wall to work out the kinks in your neck and shoulder muscles. Your restroom workout should leave you sufficiently alert to withstand another hour of boredom.

Stash a squishy ball or your favorite pet rock in your briefcase and take it out at the start of the meeting to roll between your hands or play with. Don't forget to bring a pen and legal pad to take notes and doodle during slow points.

It may also help to get up and move around a little. If it's a two-hour meeting with no intermission, prepare to excuse yourself after an hour and go for a quick walk, if only to get your blood moving.

If you can't make a getaway to the restroom or if the meeting is too formal for you to play with a ball or doodle, try wiggling your toes, twirling your ankles, and flexing your feet to stay alert. As long as your feet are under the table, no one will be the wiser!

Should I Tell My Boss
I Have Adult ADHD?

Many ADHD adults struggle over whether to tell colleagues and superiors they have the disorder. There are basically two schools of thought when it comes to disclosing your disorder in the workplace: "don't ask, don't tell" and "honesty is the best policy."

Don't Ask, Don't Tell

Some ADHD experts, pointing to the all-too-real possibility of discrimination or prejudice in the workplace, believe the "don't ask, don't tell" policy works best for many ADHD adults, especially those who have mild symptoms that are well-managed by medication.

Of course, not telling a supervisor you have a medical condition can backfire if you "cover up" your symptoms with lies or misleading statements, or if you accept a written job description of duties you know will be difficult to achieve because of your symptoms. If your undisclosed symptoms interfere with your ability to perform the job, there's a chance you could be terminated for failing to tell your boss you have adult ADHD.

Honesty Is the Best Policy

Other experts believe it's better to disclose your disorder. You may be eligible for legal protection offered by the Americans with Disabilities Act, which could protect you against discrimination because of your disabilities.

The ADA could also help you qualify for special accommodations at work or in the work environment to compensate for your ADHD symptoms. For instance, if you suffer from distractibility, you may be moved from a cubicle to a private office or be permitted to use headsets or white noise machines to eliminate noise. Or, you may be permitted to trade jobs with another employee or move to a vacant position to do a job that is a better fit for you.

Fact

While ADHD adults can enjoy some workplace protection from the ADA, the law doesn't guarantee that you'll get the job you desire or that you won't be fired for underperforming. Because the law is extremely complex, it's very difficult for an ADHD adult to sue an employer for discrimination and win under the ADA.

Another reason it may simply make sense to disclose your disorder is that many companies require the full disclosure of health issues before hiring, either for security or health insurance coverage purposes. Failing to tell a prospective employer you have adult ADHD could be grounds for not hiring you or for termination.

Your Legal Rights at Work

According to Tim Whisman, a Pasadena, California, attorney who specializes in Social Security Disability Insurance, it is indeed possible to obtain benefits for adult ADHD.

Getting an Overview of Disability

Whisman advises that you consult a lawyer if you feel your ADHD makes it impossible for you to do your job: "Your goal at this point is to get an overview of the disability application and determination process. This is not vital to your eventually obtaining benefits, but is generally a good idea so that you will know what to expect."

Learning Your Rights as an ADHD Adult

Whisman cautions that it's important to understand the criteria for disability since Social Security Disability Insurance is generally awarded to those who cannot hold down any type of job. You probably won't qualify if you can still perform another full-time job but can no longer complete the work from your prior job.

He adds, "In addition to learning about the process, you may be advised, for example, to begin documenting your problem. This may be a good time for you to begin seeking treatment for your adult ADHD because a record of evaluation and treatment will likely help substantiate your claim of disability."

Should I Hire an Attorney from the Start?

Whisman says it's probably not a good idea for you to hire an attorney or advocate at the start. Your claim may be accepted without argument and you will have to pay your attorney a portion of the award. If more information is needed before a decision can be reached, you may be sent to a doctor at no cost to you. The results of this evaluation will be used with the information you've already provided.

What If My Application Is Turned Down?

If your first application is turned down, you may ask for reconsideration, says Whisman. There is a strict time limit for appealing, and an appeal will consider the information from your original claim as well as any new evidence you can present. "Be sure to read any denial notice sent to you from the Social Security Administration carefully," Whisman advises. "If your application is turned down at this reconsideration stage and you still wish to pursue your claim, you may want to hire an attorney or other representative to help you prepare your appeal. Pay attention to time limits for filing the appeal."

The Benefits of Legal Help

Whisman says after your application is turned down, a legal hearing may be held before an administrative law judge. "At this point, hiring a representative often makes financial sense, although appeals can be successful without the involvement of a representative," he says.

Fact

An experienced attorney or representative will be able to help you get the most benefit from your medical records and will help you tell the judge the most compelling aspects of your history and circumstances, Whisman says. "This help comes at a price, but only if you win, and the price is likely worth it."

Whisman says that while his firm has seen many people win their cases without an attorney or representative, "we've also seen that many people have little idea of what is going on during their hearing, and little knowledge of how to make their cases. An experienced representative can help you deal with that."

CHAPTER 20

Finding the Silver Lining of Adult ADHD

The three major symptoms of adult ADHD create many challenges. But these symptoms may also have a silver lining. Hyperactivity can give you energy to work longer, impulsivity can prompt you to take leaps of faith, and inattention can make it easier to move between projects.

The Upside of Adult ADHD

Adult ADHD doesn't have to be a curse for life.

The New Definition of Adult ADHD

As researchers discover more and more about the disorder, they are redefining what it means to be an ADHD adult and finding the many positive traits that come with the negative ones.

Scientists believe that one reason ADHD adults may excel at creative tasks is that their brains are wired in a way that limits inhibition. ADHD adults may find it easier to follow the beat of their own drummers than non-ADHD adults who feel compelled to conform to societal norms.

Wired for the Twenty-First Century

The ADHD adult is wired for peak performance and success in the complicated and ever-changing twenty-first century.

Poised for a New Millennium

True, an ADHD adult may have problems focusing on things that are mundane and boring, such as where he put his glasses. But because their thinking process is different from that of other people, they have the sort of creative mindset that leads to great works of art, science, and invention; a surplus of ideas; great enthusiasm and excitement; prolonged interest; and the ability to see the big picture.

Right-Brain Masters

ADHD adults have the skills and right-brain power required to succeed in the twenty-first century. Because they thrive on visual imagery and stimulation, they are naturally attracted to computers, which are accelerating the rate at which new information and knowledge can be disseminated and interrelated.

Natural Entrepreneurs

Mavericks by nature, ADHD adults may not always be good followers, but they often excel as leaders.

Fact

While chronic disorganization and clutter are problems that affect most ADHD adults, many are highly adept at functioning in chaotic environments. In fact, they may actually require chaos to create, invent, or function at their peak.

If your company is stifling your creativity and motivation and you want to make a switch, consider looking for a business that is flexible and open to dialogue, where you'll have some freedom to arrange your environment, schedule, and work habits. If you're restless and unfocused at work because the issues you deal with just don't interest you, you may excel doing the exact same job if you find topics you enjoy. If your job is so stressful that you can't focus or concentrate because you're always upset, take that as a sign you need to think about making a change.

Tapping into Special ADHD Gifts

The brain chemistry of ADHD adults differs from "normal" brains in its relationship to dopamine. As a result, ADHD adults crave stimulation just to feel alive. Because of this craving, they are also more likely to seek thrills, take risks, discover new ways of doing things, act and think more boldly, stand out from the pack, and have a higher degree of personal charisma.

 Alert

If you have ADHD, you're 300 times as likely to start your own business as adults without the disorder, according to *Fortune* magazine. That's because ADHD adults are more likely to take risks than others, and many of them also prefer working for themselves. Because they have the courage to take chances, many ADHD adults become self-made millionaires.

If you have adult ADHD, you may already have the raw material it takes to gain great fame and wealth. But why does the ADHD gene help a few people achieve outrageous success while leaving many others struggling just to get by? While luck and chance always play some role, the real secret may lie in understanding how to harness your innate strengths and minimize your ADHD weaknesses.

Harnessing Your ADHD Strengths

One of the most important things you can do to maximize your strengths is to manage your adult ADHD symptoms consistently and effectively.

Essential

Take your medication regularly. While medication alone can't fix a flagging career or make the wrong career feel right, it can help you manage mood swings and alleviate restlessness and bad temper while you're in the process of looking or preparing for a new career.

For most ADHD adults, the best treatment approach is a combination of medication, therapy, behavioral modification, healthy eating habits, regular exercise, support groups, relaxation techniques, and other lifestyle changes that enhance your life.

How to Make Adult ADHD Work for You

In addition to following your treatment program, you can turn many of your ADHD symptoms into assets by using the following tips and strategies.

- Don't repress your adult ADHD gifts. Instead, look for ways to express your creativity, inventiveness, imagination, enthusiasm, and energy at work, at home, and in social settings.
- Let your inattention be your guide. If you find your mind constantly drifting and wandering, don't ignore the danger signs. Inattention can be a red flag that you're bored, disinterested, or unchallenged. ADHD can be the radar you need to switch to a new career. For instance, if your job is stifling you and making you feel depressed, lethargic, and brain-dead, it may be another indication that it's time for a job switch. If you're in a job that you find boring, mundane, or

uninteresting, you'll have difficulty applying your ADHD hyperfocus and creativity to tasks and probably daydream or zone out instead.

- Make a list of your strengths and weaknesses, and then make a second list of all the jobs and careers you've had. Match up your strengths and weaknesses to the various jobs to get a better idea of what types of work you're best suited for.

- If you're not sure how to best use your ADHD skills, or if you're not even sure what they are, talk to a career coach or therapist. Aptitude tests can help you hone in on jobs and careers that will set your brain cells firing.

- Remember that ambition alone is not enough to propel you to success. Many ADHD adults find it easy to get enthused about a new career but aren't realistic about the time and effort required to get there. Create a road map to get you from point A to point B, then use your tremendous energy and drive to propel you down the road to success, step by manageable step.

- Take inventory of your personal likes and dislikes. Do you like working on your feet in front of people (like a teacher) or by yourself in front of a computer (like a writer)? If you're hyperactive, you might fare best in a job that lets you move around, such as a sales job that gets you out and about, or a career that requires physical exertion, such as a personal trainer.

- Don't stick with a job that doesn't match your personal profile just because you've worked extra hard to master it or worked against some of your natural gifts or characteristics to be successful. You'll be happier, less stressed, and more effective at a job that uses your natural gifts.

- Test drive another career. If your current job is not using your imagination or creativity to the fullest, make arrangements to shadow someone whose career you admire. For more information, visit *www.vocationvacations.com*.

- Be patient with yourself. Don't expect to go from the wrong job to the absolute perfect job in one easy step. Prepare to spend some time examining your talents and skills, talking with professionals, test driving new careers, or even going back to school to learn the skills for a new profession.

Flying Solo

If you decide to be your own boss or start your own company, make sure to hire people who complement you. If you're a big-picture person who doesn't have the patience for details, hire someone who enjoys handling what you might find boring. On the other hand, if you aren't comfortable interacting with others, hire a public relations director to handle publicity.

When You're the Boss

If you plan to start your own business and hire others to help you, you should also be aware of how your adult ADHD symptoms may affect your ability to work with employees and consider the following stumbling blocks. If they all sound like you and you're still determined to run your own business, you may want to hire a company psychotherapist and/or a second-in-command with a more affable personality to handle office snafus and miscommunications.

- ❏ Many ADHD adults find it difficult to delegate work to others, believing they are the only ones capable of dealing with it.
- ❏ Because ADHD bosses are often capable of working very long hours and hyperfocusing intently for long periods of time, they may be overly demanding employers who are unrealistic about what their employees can accomplish in a given time.

❏ ADHD adults tend to be very impatient, intolerant, and critical—traits that can quickly undermine and discourage employees.

❏ Because of their tendency to think quickly, think outside the box, and make associations between seemingly unrelated concepts or ideas, many ADHD bosses can sound like they're speaking a foreign language to employees. Their tendency to speak rapidly and leave thoughts hanging in midair may also contribute to miscommunication and frustration in the workplace.

❏ ADHD adults have notoriously short tempers and a lack of patience, and may come across as tyrants and/or control freaks to employees.

The Importance of Owning Up

Many ADHD adults have become adept at masking their symptoms or covering them up with learned behavior. While masking negative symptoms can certainly help life go more smoothly, masking positive traits such as creativity, spontaneity, or unconventional thinking could limit your ability to live your life to the fullest.

If you're in denial about your adult ADHD symptoms and/or you've been masquerading as a "normal" person out of fear of societal stigmas, it may be time to let your ADHD genie out of the box. Your therapist can help you "own" your positive ADHD traits and come up with ways to use them to their best advantage.

Harnessing the Power of Friendship

Deciding whether or not to tell friends you have adult ADHD could have a major effect on the way friends interact with and support you, and it may also impact feelings of trust.

⊡ Essential

> If your symptoms are so mild that they don't interfere with your ability to make and keep friends or if your symptoms are controlled by medication, telling your friends you have adult ADHD is probably a decision you'll make on a case-by-case, or need-to-know, basis.

If your symptoms result in periodic moodiness, irritability, withdrawing, socially awkward behavior (like putting your foot in your mouth), a tendency toward reckless behavior, impatience, or restlessness, you may want to inform close friends. This way, they will be more understanding of your symptoms, better able to put your ADHD-inspired idiosyncrasies into perspective, and more forgiving when you say or do something inappropriate.

Capitalizing on Role Models

Close friends can help you avoid embarrassing faux pas and help you function more effectively in social settings. They can act as your personal interpreter when you can't follow a conversation, lose track of your thoughts, or are unable to read nonverbal cues or body language.

Friends who have also been diagnosed with adult ADHD can be an indispensable support system. Whether it's providing a safe place for you to rant about your symptoms or discussing the latest information on ADHD resources, these friends can offer the support, sympathy, and empathy you need to coexist peacefully with adult ADHD.

The Future of Adult ADHD

Although scientists have yet to find a cure for adult ADHD, high-tech research and equipment are shedding new light on the disorder's causes and potential treatments.

Many researchers now believe that adult ADHD is not one condition but a cluster of conditions or disorders, each of which may be treatable. By discovering treatments for the individual conditions that make up adult ADHD, scientists one day hope to find an overall cure for the disorder.

Ever-Evolving Research

The rapidly evolving technology of brain-imaging techniques is letting scientists observe how the ADHD brain functions. By comparing ADHD brains to conventional brains, they are finding distinctive differences in brain chemistry and makeup that categorize ADHD. Scientists are hopeful that brain-imaging techniques can one day be used in the diagnosis and subsequent management of ADHD.

Better Criteria for Better Diagnoses

The current criteria for the diagnosis of ADHD are taken from the *Diagnostic and Statistical Manual of Mental Health Disorders, 4th edition* (*DSM-IV*), which was published in 1994.

The next edition will be published in 2013 and will reflect current research findings. Researchers are pushing for modifications in the 2013 edition that would establish different diagnostic criteria for childhood, adolescent, and adult ADHD.

New Directions in Research

Researchers are studying the long-term effects of established ADHD treatments, such as medication, psychotherapy, and behavioral modification, and are also looking at the long-term outcome of ADHD children who are not diagnosed or treated.

In addition, scientists are looking for safer and more effective medications to treat patients with ADHD alone, and those with ADHD and co-existing conditions such as chronic anxiety, depression, and bipolar disorder.

Closing in on the Mysteries

Although there is no cure for adult ADHD on the immediate horizon, scientists are closing in on the mysteries behind this elusive disorder. Less than twenty years ago, many people, including top scientists, regarded ADHD as a fictional disorder used to justify bad behavior, or a behavior problem caused by lax parenting. Very few people had even heard of adult ADHD.

Alert

Today, many researchers believe that adult ADHD is a neurobiological disorder or a cluster of different disorders caused by a chemical imbalance of multiple neurotransmitters in the brain. The key players are believed to be dopamine, norepinephrine, and serotonin.

While no one can promise that a cure for adult ADHD will be found in your lifetime, rapid advances in technology and a heightened awareness of ADHD mean the chances of that happening have never been better.

Symptoms Checklist

Use the following checklists for reference as you increase your understanding of the symptoms associated with adult ADHD. Note the symptoms you may be suffering from, and be sure to explain them to your physician.

Personal and Family History Symptoms

- Personal history of ADHD symptoms in childhood that include inattention, hyperactivity, impulsivity, distraction, restlessness, and disorganization
- Family history of ADHD as well as chronic depression, anxiety, bipolar disorder, or substance or alcohol abuse in parents, siblings, or relatives
- History of not meeting your potential at school, in college, and in the workplace, as noted on report cards, exams, and job performance reviews
- History of behavior problems at home, at school, and at work, including chronic lateness, delinquency, and behavior requiring disciplinary action
- History of bedwetting past the age of five years old

Symptoms of Inattention
- Inability to stay focused on material unless you have a high interest in it
- Easily distracted
- Tendency to drift or wander when subject is boring or dull
- Tendency to hyperfocus on interesting material to the exclusion of everything else
- Failure to focus or pay attention to details and "fine print"
- Inability to follow written or spoken directions
- Inability to track or follow extended conversations
- Tendency to forget where you put things
- Difficulty learning new skills because of an inability to pay attention and stay on track
- Difficulty staying on track while reading
- Inability to stay focused during sexual intimacy
- Tendency to drift off or tune out when uninterested or bored
- Inability to listen carefully

Symptoms of Impulsivity
- Tendency to engage in impulsive behavior such as impulsive spending, gambling, driving, drinking, substance abuse, illicit sex, and eating
- Prone to interrupting conversations and blurting out inappropriate or irrelevant comments
- Tendency to speak before thinking and put foot in mouth
- Inability to follow established chains of command, proper procedures, regulations, rules, and bylaws
- Feeling impatient, rushed, and like there's never enough time
- Low tolerance for frustration
- Tendency to be tactless and overly blunt
- Tendency to change or quit jobs frequently and impulsively
- Prone to lying, exaggerating, and making grandiose promises you can't keep
- Tendency to shop-lift and steal

Symptoms of Hyperactivity
- Inability to sit still for periods of time
- Tendency to abuse caffeine, alcohol, and drugs to self-medicate
- Short temper and outbursts of rage
- Oversensitive to comments and criticism
- Overly critical
- Constant search for thrills, excitement, and stimulation (gambling, drugs, alcohol, sex, racing, etc.)
- Tendency to be pick fights or start arguments
- Prone to obsessive worrying and fretting
- Prone to addictive behaviors such as drinking, substance abuse, gambling, and sex
- Tendency to talk incessantly, monopolize conversations, boast, and brag
- Performance worsens under pressure
- Tendency to "go blank" during tests

Symptoms of Restlessness
- Tendency to constantly fidget and doodle
- Trouble sitting still in one place for long periods of time
- Inability to think unless in motion
- Feeling extremely restless for no specific reason
- Feeling anxious and nervous for no specific reason

Symptoms of Disorganization
- Inability to plan ahead
- Trouble prioritizing and dividing large projects into smaller tasks
- Prone to clutter, piles, and leaving a mess behind
- Prone to chronic procrastination, lateness, feelings of being rushed
- Inability to meet deadlines
- Tendency toward clutter and messiness

- Easily overwhelmed by everyday things in life
- Unable to manage, control, and track personal and family finances
- Problems getting started and following through
- Scattered and frenzied thinking

Workplace Symptoms

- Symptoms of disorganization
- Tendency to be a workaholic
- Tendency to work late or take work home because of inability to meet deadlines and focus at work
- Poor work history. Tendency to be demoted, dismissed, and disciplined
- Problems dealing with bosses, superiors, and authority figures
- Tendency to earn much less than peers
- Tendency to underperform, regardless of ability or potential
- Prone to disregarding rules, regulations, and policies
- Tendency toward chronic lateness or absenteeism

Physical Symptoms

- Difficulty with hand-eye coordination in sports like baseball, football, golf, and tennis
- Poor or illegible handwriting
- Problems expressing information
- Chronic fidgeting, squirming, repetitive habits, and tics
- Insomnia due to racing thoughts; inability to fall asleep or stay asleep
- Problems waking up
- Wildly fluctuating mood and energy swings
- Feeling sleepy or tired during the day
- Hypersensitive to touch, sounds, smells, light, clothing, jewelry
- Tendency to scare or startle easily
- Tendency toward over-exercising

Interpersonal and Relationship Symptoms
- Inability to make and keep meaningful relationships
- Inability to establish intimacy during sex
- Tendency to forget important times and dates
- Tendency to engage in extramarital affairs to find excitement and thrills
- High incidence of separation, divorce, and child custody suits
- Inability to stay focused and perform during sexual activities

Symptoms in Social Settings
- Feeling socially awkward and uncomfortable in social settings
- Tendency to frustrate and alienate friends and family members
- Feeling isolated, alone, and like a social outcast
- Tendency to prefer being alone to social interaction

Additional Resources

Organizations/Support Groups

Children and Adults with Attention-Deficit/Hyperactivity Disorder (CHADD)

A nonprofit organization and support group for children and adults with ADHD.

www.chadd.org

National Attention Deficit Disorder Association (ADDA)

A national organization for adults with ADHD with conferences and teleclasses.

www.add.org

National ADHD Service

A national organization with a provider directory and free resources on ADHD.

www.addresources.org

National Center for Gender Issues and ADHD

An advocacy group that promotes research and awareness on ADHD in women and girls.

www.ncgiadd.org

ADDvance

An online resource network for parents, teens, young adults, adults, women and girls.
www.addvance.com

Books

Barkley, Russell, Murphy, Kevin, and Mariellen Fischer. *ADHD in Adults, What the Science Says* (New York: The Guilford Press, 2008).

Shapiro, Joan, M.D., and Jeffrey Freed. *4 Weeks to an Organized Life with AD/HD* (New York: Taylor Trade Publishing, 2007).

Adler, Lenard, *Scattered Minds* (New York: G.P. Putnam, 2006).

Hallowell, Edward and John Ratey. *Delivered from Distraction* (New York: Ballatine, 2005).

Brown, Thomas. *Attention Deficit Disorder: The Unfocused Mind in Children and Adults* (New Haven: Yale University Press, 2005).

Matlin, Terry. *Survival Tips for Women with AD/HD* (Plantation, Fla: Specialty Press, 2005).

Adem, Daniel. *Healing the Hardware of the Soul* (New York: Free Press, 2002).

Adamec, Christine. *Moms with ADD* (Dallas: Taylor Trade Publishing, 2000).

Hallowell, Edward, and John Ratey. *Answers to Distraction* (New York: Bantam Books, 1996).

Hallowell, Edward, and John Ratey. *Driven to Distraction* (New York: Simon and Schuster, 1994).

Websites

ADD.about.com

This site is a great introduction to ADHD in children and adults.
www.add.about.com

Additude Magazine.com

This is a free website covering most aspects of ADHD in adults and children.
www.additudemag.com

ADD Forums

This website is an online support network for adults, teens, and parents.
www.addforums.com

ADHD News.com

This is a support and information website for adults and children with ADHD.

www.adhdnews.com

ADD Consults.com

This online virtual clinic offers free one-on-one advice from ADHD experts.

www.addconsults.com

Index

A

B